1

To:

From:

Date:

Message:

Dedication

There are people you meet in life that change the way you think about the others you've met in life. People who prove to you that some individuals are worth trusting and allowing into your life. The special ones who can alter your entire perspective on life itself. Alison is one of those people, and she also talked me into writing this book.

This book is dedicated to my college Professor Alison. I wish there were more people like you! Thank you for everything you do for everyone!

Introduction

In this book I claim no special authority for the opinions I have and the things I believe in. This book is a simple explanation of how we live that works for us. The way we live may not work for everyone else.

I am quite an opinionated person and enjoy sharing what it is I feel. Be that right or wrong, which you'll soon read... it's a southern thing.

Whether my beliefs are scientifically proven or not, I will still believe just what it is I believe. This is my somewhat comedic version of living on a small farm, the silly and serious ways we figure things out, and how much fun we have though we work so damn hard for what we have.

I wouldn't trade the way we live for anything, not voluntarily anyway.

Contents

Chapter 1
How We Got Started

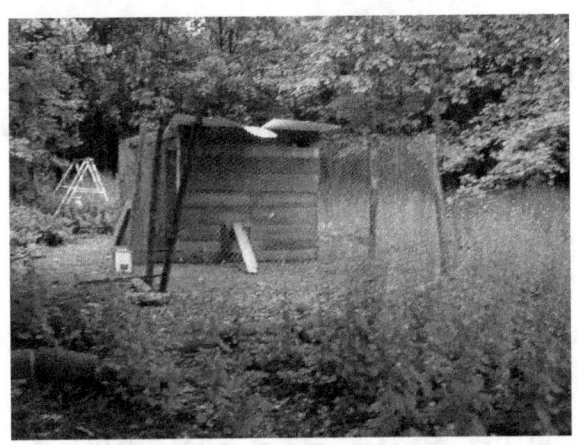

{This is a side view of the chicken coop with the outside pen. At this time it was almost completed, but lacked a couple details to be finished.}

When my husband Joseph and I first started out, we weren't much different than many others who didn't come from money. Our house was in need of much repair and maintenance and he was paying child support. Our vehicles were getting older and also needing repairs. To say we had a budget was more of a joke than a possibility. No matter how I figured it we would always be way short on covering our expenses. We were stuck in a revolving "rob Peter to pay Paul" scenario.

Through Joseph's work and my work we would sometimes get the opportunity to clean up "garbage" at people's job-sites and sometimes from their houses. Occasionally someone would call with free wood if we cut it down or picked it up.

When I moved in with Joseph there was a small wood stove in the living room which heated the whole house. With my little truck or the wheel barrow we would bring wood to the house and stack what we could fit in the living room and on the front porch. What we could fit would usually last for about four to six days depending on how cold it got. It was funny too because a lot of our friends said I wouldn't last one year in this kind of environment. It didn't take long for me to give up on keeping lotion in our bedroom; once it freezes it's never the same. It's interesting to look back now and realize just how little my friends actually knew about me. I have carried a knife in my pocket since I was in high school. I was/am a true farm kid. I have never been much of a material person. I was lathered with material things as a child, but they were never an obsession of mine. Me and Joseph became the perfect fit for each other.

I adjusted rather well to giving up certain silly luxuries. I never like any of that lotion for your face anyway, makes me feel greasy and dirty. Once those trivial things were gone, I didn't really seem to miss them much.

The biggest adjustment was not having money for groceries and the electricity bill. It always managed to come down to one or the other, and the electricity bill usually won unfortunately. So it became quite a treat to take the trailer and head out for a garbage clean up mission. We couldn't afford to go shopping and at least we could end up with something we didn't already have and those little missions became our mock shopping sprees.

One of our first few clean up missions included these crates that were about six feet wide and about eight feet tall. Only one was in good enough shape for use, the other was spare wood. We also ended up with some old left over silt fence. For those of you who aren't familiar with what silt fence is, it's what you see around construction sites to contain the soil from running off into the roadways or sewers.

Where we live, our property is split in three different sections. It is set rather strange, but we can live with it. We live on about seventy acres which is surrounded by houses and apartments now. It used to be like living in our own little world with only a few lights edging our property reminding us of the outside world. A world we try not to think about, especially with how bad the people have become where we are. I really wish there weren't so many people moving in all around us. There is nothing worse to me than living in the city. Someone is always in your business. That just isn't the way southerners where we come from are raised. I can't figure out why all these new people moving out here from the city think our property is there to trespass on and steal from as they see fit. Where we come from, if you don't own it you stay the hell off it!

I'm sure we aren't the only ones who have this problem either. For many years now people have been pouring in to what used to be a quiet and calm country atmosphere. Where we live not so very long ago was nothing but farms and farmers fields.

As the people from the city have moved out here by the hundreds, many of them began to complain about the smell of the cows, pigs and horses. They complained about the farm equipment on the roads, and blatantly trespass and shine deer right in front of our house. I'm not saying everyone from the city is like that, but I have to say that the majority of them have been.

It hasn't mattered how old they are either. I have seen more than four grown adults walk into our flower beds and start ripping our flowers up by the roots, right in front of me and while I was yelling at them to get the hell out of my flowers! Then they act like they have no clue why I would be mad. Hello? I would never walk into someone's yard and get into their flowers, not to mention think of stealing them! That should give you a very small window into the kind of crap we have dealing with from these kinds of people for years now. With each passing year they seem to only get worse.

That being said maybe you now have an idea why Joseph and I enjoy the seclusion of where we live, and why we miss the way things used to be so much.

Joseph and I both grew up on small farms when we were younger. We were both raised around hunting and we also ate our "pets". Though our cattle and livestock were never intended to be pets, they always ended up being just that anyway. We both accepted the natural order of things at a young age and had no qualms about the way things were meant to be by living the way those who came before us did. We were well aware that when we sat down to dinner we were eating something or everything that we had raised ourselves. We were both part of a whole family who got off our butts and went and helped around our small family farms.

When we got together we started reminiscing about our childhoods and missing our gardens and chickens. The difference in eating farm fresh meat, we could talk about that for hours and dream of winning the lottery so we could continue that tradition.

When we ended up with the over sized crates from our clean up mission, we had big plans. The plan was to build a chicken coop. Across the road there used to be a barn which by now has fallen down. The old barn still has some good wood to be gleaned from it, and there is where we began the new chicken coop. We cut barn wood for the floor of the coop, and it looked better than the wood floor in our dining room! We went on to grab and cut more barn wood to build three sides of the coop. For the final side we re-used a door from the barn that still has an original piece of old hardware that we still use for the handle to open the door today. The hinges were also original and are still holding up the door as well as opening and closing the door today. They just don't make things like they used to.

We went to the home improve-
ment store and purchased several
sheets of white corrugated plastic
roofing panels. We had to buy the
cheapest ones they had because we
were broke. We got a couple tubes of
silicone and used that to seal the screw
holes from where we attached the
panels to the roof of our new chicken
coop. We cut a hole in one side of the
coop wall, closer to the ground, and we
built a little hatch door that folded
down and doubled as a ramp when it
was open. I found a couple hinges
floating around the house and used
those to secure the hatch door to the
coop wall on the outside. I bought a
latch at the dollar store to hold the little
door closed at night to keep the critters
out and the chickens in. I even added
the little boards on the inside of that
little door which reminded me of
Foghorn Leghorn and the dog from the
old Bugs Bunny cartoons we grew up

with. The chicken coop in the cartoon is where I got the idea to make those cute little steps on the hatch door. In all reality they didn't turn out to be very functional little boards, but it was my silent amusement of thinking about Foghorn Leghorn that made me smile when I looked at it. It gave me a feeling of accomplishment.

We used more old barn wood to build nests into the wall of the inside of the chicken coop. We ended up with two columns side by side that go from the bottom of the coop to the top. About six nests per column, or twelve in all. We got some free scrap fencing and ended up using that to make an outside pen for the future chickens. They would need to be able to get outside to get sunlight and fresh air for times when they couldn't be let out. The posts for the outside pen were four small trees that needed to be cut down anyway. Those four trees were set just as you would set poles for any other fence. Joseph used the chain saw to clean any branches off before we set them in their intended places. Joseph spent many very hot hours in the summer sun with a pair of post hole diggers trying to get through the clay which to me seemed to be as hard as concrete. I felt bad watching him do all the hard work and wanted to help. I told him to take a break and let me dig for a little while. When I tried, I thought I was hitting rocks. I couldn't get anything out of the hole. When he took the post hole diggers back and came up with more dirt I couldn't believe it! I wasn't used to feeling that helpless, but helpless in that situation I certainly was.

With all of the poles set for the outside pen, the fencing fun began. We put one section up and attached part of that section to the coop itself so that no critter could get through it and get to the future chickens. I wasn't working for the rest of the end of that summer, I had been laid off, and Joseph seemed to do nothing but have to work. So, I took it upon myself to finish the fencing and what was left to do in the chicken coop. The fencing was chain link and ten feet tall. It was very heavy and very awkward to maneuver by ones-self. I somehow managed to drag, push, pull, and curse enough to get it all attached. I even managed to put the pieces on the top and attach that as well to complete the cover over the outside pen. That was by far the worst part! I spent half my time on a ladder with the fencing resting on my head, but I was determined to get it done. There were some areas that were a little short where there was still a gap in the fencing. We almost had enough to complete the pen, but not quite. I went back over to the old barn and started hunting for some old chicken wire or old fencing. I found some and used what I could to start covering any gaps that were left in the fencing. We ended up buying a small role of chicken wire and I finished the gaps in the fence with the new chicken wire and some mechanics wire I had gotten at a garage sale for about twenty-five cents. I weaved the mechanics wire through the fencing patches, just like you would if you were sewing. This ended up making a very strong mend, stronger than I had expected. Finally, we were ready for chickens!

During this chicken coop building excursion we did everything by hand or with hand tools. We carried the wood from one side of the road to the other while we were working on the coop. The extent of our tools were very basic. I used left over screws and nails, and anything else I could find to keep the job going without having to buy anything. When you don't have money and you want something bad enough, you'll figure a way to get it done. It took longer than most coops would have taken these days if you have money for augers and other luxuries that make jobs much easier. But think about how much exercise and working out we got from that project. That may not have been the intention, but it is what happens around a farm. None of our friends helped us; it was just me and Joseph. We worked our asses off making something out of nothing because we were poor. Spending time together like that might not be the way some people would refer to quality time, but it was and still is for us. Events like these can bring you closer to each other. Especially when realize the only people you can depend on is each other.

That summer, and that chicken coop, is where everything Joseph and I were to become with one another began. We found our roots together and started building on all of the things we started out with when we were young. Getting back to basics I guess you could call it, and desperately in search of better food to put on the table. We didn't have much by most people's standards. The way we seen it we had more than most, and were very proud to have built it with our very own hands, blood, sweat and beers as I like to refer to it.

When we started out we had no idea that we would learn so much from almost everything we did. We both began looking to our pasts for answers to how our parents did things when we were growing up. We were hoping we would be able to remember enough from our farming childhoods to make a success out of all the things we had planned.

Chapter 2
Getting Started Stories

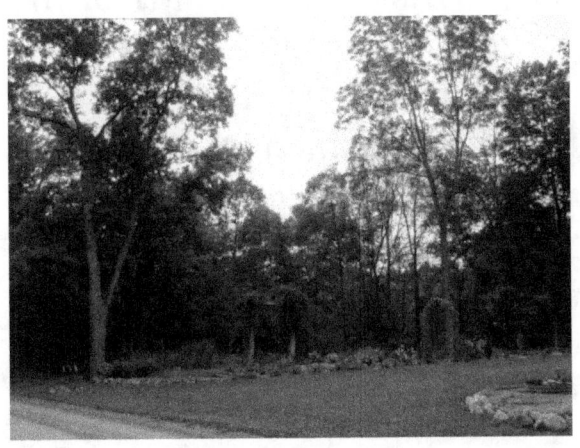

{This picture gives you an idea of a portion of the flower beds we have put in.}

When I first moved in with Joseph he had been single for several years I guess. The bachelor life did not include home décor. Which that should, for the most part, go without saying. I don't mean that in a bad way. There really aren't a great deal of men who seem to care about keeping a clean and neat house, or that the curtains match the furniture. That is usually what women are known for, though I know not all men or women are exactly like that.

There weren't many functional things around his house. At first I could barely get into the driveway because the driveway closely resembled a mud bog. Which is just fine under the right circumstances, just not in front of the main entrance to the house. Driving an S-10 did not work very well, he had a big four wheel drive, so naturally he could have cared less about the driveway. If I could have afforded a big four wheel drive, I probably wouldn't have cared about the driveway either. None the less, shortly after I moved in Joseph began to put in an actual driveway. He dug up all of the soil and hauled in a base for the new driveway. After he leveled the base he capped it with another load or two of smaller stone. While that job was in progress he lined our horseshoe driveway with boulders that we hauled in. None of that was cheap, and we were barely able to get that done. We skipped a few bills here and there, but it was worth it. Now, not only did we have a functional driveway, but we also had another spot for flowers. We hauled in topsoil that was suitable for flowers. With a rake and a shovel, I ended up leveling out the five yards of topsoil in the area in the middle of the driveway. I surprised Joseph with that when he came home the next day, he couldn't believe that I had it finished by myself. He was working so much that I didn't want him to come home and have all of that to contend with. His job can be very physically demanding.

I think I put in just as many hours that summer working on the house and the yard as Joseph did at his job. Most of the yard work was Joseph's area, but I helped with whatever it was I could do. He was (and still is) the brains and the brawn of any outdoor operation that we get involved in. He is very good at that sort of thing, and our yard proves it.

The middle of the driveway was to be the "wild flower" area. No mulch, no plan, just colorful flowers everywhere of every size, shape, and color. Well, the plan started off with good intentions, but there was not enough sunlight to sprout the idea into reality. We bought so many seed packets and had menial results with most of them. Most of the seeds we had wanted to plant required more sunlight than the area we put them in could provide. I ended up buying a bunch of plants I found one sale to put in so we would at least have something. That is until one of the neighbors in the nearby sub division came along and let her dog run all over the newly transplanted plants and then peed all over them. She and her dog killed about fifty dollars worth of plants.

Now with a few more trees gone, these days it is beginning to look more like we had planned it to look in the beginning stages of its creation. Joseph has a green thumb and anything he touches when it comes to plants, or anything in nature for that matter, flourishes. He has a special connection with the natural world that I find fascinating.

Between him and I, there is virtually nothing we can't accomplish together. After I finished painting and stripping old wallpaper inside the house; making the house "prettier".

Better yet, how about livable, I think that would better describe all the inside work that needed to be done around the house. If I remember correctly, it took me about three months to clean the house up. Everything had to be organized, painted, and a great deal of old clutter just needed to be thrown away. After the house was finally finished, we went back to focusing on work in the yard, not that Joseph ever really stopped. He was always finding something new to spruce up or create around the yard.

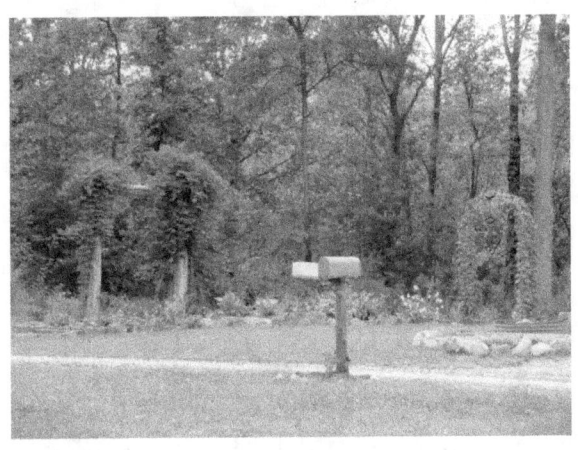

{You might be able to see the trellis on the left which used to be two trees, the one on the right Joseph made from our scrap pile.}

We spent the rest of that summer and a couple more summers making an actual yard area and taking down trees that were threats to the house. After quite a bit of clearing to make a yard area, we commenced to creating some beautiful flower beds. There has been at least one flower bed or flower area created almost every year since we have been together. All of those areas have been constructed with nothing more than wheel barrows and shovels. Of course, a couple rakes as well. We aren't talking about small flower beds either. Everything Joseph does is well thought out and as elaborate as we can physically handle to make it. As well as what we can afford or find for topsoil. Everything we have built together has been built by hand and one piece at a time. We are still hoping one day to be able to invest in a piece of equipment of some sort to make things a little easier. No, a lot easier because we sure aren't getting any younger.

For the two of us, there seems to be nothing we can't accomplish when we put our hearts and heads together to make it happen. In all things we do, it takes both of us giving one hundred percent or these dreams would never have had a chance to even begin to materialize. Not as much as they have to this point at least.

The first couple winters and summers Joseph and I lived together were kind of crazy in several aspects. One thing that really stands out in my mind is a tree that was only a foot or two off from the side of the house. This tree had been there for many, many years and had probably been dying for several years or more. I can't remember now what kind of tree it was, a hard maple I think, but it stood at least sixty to seventy feet tall. The trunk was at least three feet and maybe even four feet in circumference. About ten or fifteen feet from the ground, the tree had a Y. Where the tree y'ed the two trunks that grew from that y were by no means small. When a tree does this it allows water to pool and run off in a particular area with every rain fall. These types of natural occurrences in trees can create areas where critters and ants like to begin digging in and making nests when the trees begin to get softer as they start to rot. Trees that close to the house also allow critters access to the roof of your house. There was more than one tree that close to the house, but this tree was the one I remember most because it was so scary. Most of, well all of, the bark had already fallen off of the tree by this time and the raccoons were using it to get to the roof of the house. The tree had a split that went from the Y of the tree all the way to the ground and half of the tree was leaning over the entire back half of the house. During storms or windy days, the tree had split so bad that no-one would go into the dining room or kitchen for fear of the tree falling on the house and possibly killing one of us. In a rush one day just as an ice storm was coming in. Joseph and I went out with a ladder and cabled the tree together so it would be less likely to give way and take out the house. This bought us enough time to make it to spring and then cut the tree down. To look at the tree one couldn't help but wonder how it had stayed standing for as long as it had with the condition it had been in. That was a close call.

In the spring we had to call the electric company to come out and detach the wires from our house. This tree was surrounded by a triangle of problems. Power lines on one side, the house on another side, and the lines that ran from the pole to the house on the last side. There was only one way this tree could be removed. The tree had to be cabled and pulled in only one direction or it would have been major catastrophe. I was a nervous wreck driving the truck worrying about the tree being too heavy and going backwards onto the house. Josephs truck proved to be up to the challenge and so did I. It only took us about an hour after the guy showed up to remove the wires from our house for us to cut the tree down and move it out of the way for the guy to come back and re-attach the wires to the house again.

After we had cut the tree down we noticed a couple holes that were in the upper part of the tree and not in view if you had looked up. We had looked at the tree before we cut it down to see if there were any nests, and we hadn't seen or heard anything. We were (are) always conscious of the natural world and did (still do) our best to not disturb it. After looking at the holes, it didn't appear that anything had been living in them at the time.

With the tree down for a little while we began to hear some faint chirping. We started to look around for where the noise was coming from and that is how we discovered the hole did have a nest. Apparently this was the time of year when the babies hadn't quite left the nest yet, but they were very close to doing so. We hadn't expected this because we watch the birds all the time and had never seen any birds coming or going from this tree.

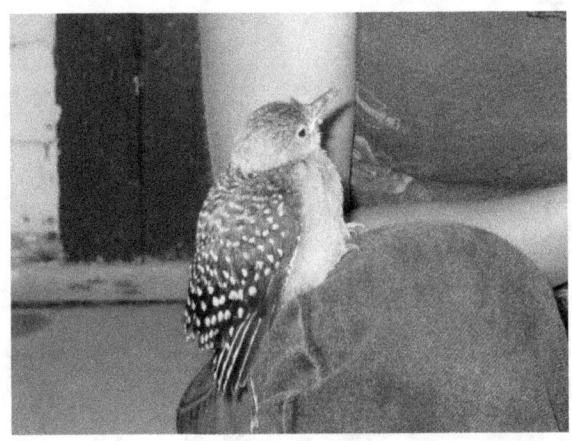

After a few minutes of following the faint little chirp we found the hole that had been at the top of the tree and had been facing the ground. We realized that was where the chirping had started coming from. I have very tiny hands and was almost able to reach in to retrieve the baby bird. We had to tip the piece of the branch up some to scoot the baby bird closer to the entrance of the hole before I could grab it. Along with the scared little bird were three of its' nest mates, and they were all dead.

I cried I felt so horrible. I felt it was our obligation to take care of this little one since we had destroyed its home and had accidentally killed its nest mates. We had an extra bird cage around and that seemed to work just fine to house our new member of our family whom we called "Woody". I spent the last money we had in our pockets on baby bird formula from the pet store and commenced to doing the best I could to give this baby a chance at survival.

Through a little internet research a few days later we learned that once you take in a woodpecker, they will never leave. If that was true I am not sure, but that is what we read. We spent a lot of time with Woody, carrying him around the yard on our shoulders. Woody would always wander all over you as you walked around and that was just too cute! Not one single time did Woody ever try to fly off or even leave our shoulders.

At the time we had not thought far enough ahead to think of exactly how long the parents feed their babies in the wild. This was no little bird, Woody was pretty big and seemed to be of an age where he could start eating more solid foods than just baby formula.

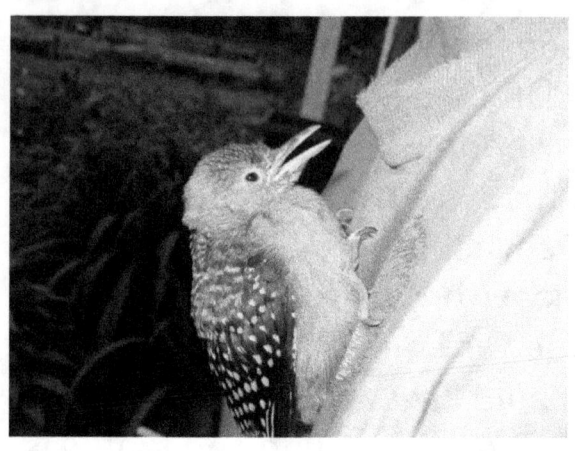

I have always been a bird lover. I find something completely fascinating about birds. They can speak in any language you teach them to, they can fly, and they are very loving and affectionate creatures for the most part. I have spent a great deal of time around baby and young birds during my lifetime as well. After about a month of having Woody, we decided to begin introducing small pieces of worms into his diet. One day Joseph and I fed Woody what would have been one whole worm about two or three inches long if you put all the pieces we fed him together. The next morning when Joseph and I got up Woody was dead on the floor of the cage. I cried, I was so sad and had assumed that we fed Woody worms to early.

We gave Woody a proper burial and swore that if we are ever put in that position again we will do more research to be sure that the baby would have a better chance to survive.

The coons on the other hand weren't so lucky. I hadn't noticed what had been going on until Joseph had pointed it out. As far as that tree was concerned, we hadn't had enough time, money, or material to handle that situation in any other way. The tree was a big problem which posed a major threat to our home and our safety.

Before the tree had been taken down, there had been other issues at hand that needed to be dealt with, issues which I had been oblivious to. Let me explain that crazy couple of months during our new lives together before the falling of that tree.

When I moved in there had been a hole in the roof next to that tree that was covered by a tarp. During all the painting and re-arranging in the house I hadn't really given it much thought. It had rained several times and I hadn't noticed anything so it wasn't at the forefront of my thoughts. I had however noticed all the noise I would hear at night. In passing I think Joseph had mentioned that before, but once again that didn't really stand out much in my mind. When I would ask what all that noise was, he would usually say it was probably the squirrels or a coon. Let me tell you if, if you don't live in a farm house, and you don't already know this, squirrels are loud! I had grown up in a farm house, and I remember hearing the squirrels run across my ceiling and through the walls every night. I just don't ever remember them being this loud.

It didn't take long before the squirrel's started sounding like a herd of elephants in the walls and the ceiling. Right about that same time I started to notice water in the kitchen when it rained one evening. When we went outside the next day to look at the roof and I couldn't believe what Joseph said to me. That a raccoon had dug its way into the house again. He said that hole that had been under that tarp had gotten there because a raccoon had literally dug into the roof to get into the attic. I have seen some shit in my day, but that was unreal. That night we had sat outside with flash lights. We waited until we started hearing all the loud noises making their way to the kitchen ceiling. That's when I seen that Joseph had been right. Not that I thought he had been lying to me. I had just found what he had said to be almost unbelievable. Something that I would have to see for myself to fully believe I suppose. When we heard the noise at the kitchen from outside in the yard where we had been sitting on the lawn, we turned on the flashlights and there it was. A giant raccoon poking its head out of the roof! This was no small hole. This hole was about two feet wide and about three or four feet long by now. It was huge! The more that raccoon had come in and out, the bigger that hole had gotten. How often have you heard someone say a raccoon is peeking out of the middle of their roof?

Needless to say we had been sitting in the yard with not just flashlights. As soon as that raccoon made its' way out of the roof and had given us a clear shot, we had taken it.

After we got rid of the raccoon we went back in the house and thought the problem had been cured. Well, it would have been. We were still hearing a lot of noise. Noise that was louder than the usual grey squirrel, red squirrel, and flying squirrel's that we were used to hearing. Yep, the damn coon had babies. It took a week, many late nights and a lot of beer to finish getting rid of all those baby coons that were living in the ceiling and walls of the house. The last one we ended up having to fish out of the wall because that is where it fell! When I say fish for it, I am not kidding, I had used a fishing pole to get the darn thing out. I was getting quite anxious to get them out of there so we could try to patch that hole in the roof before it rained anymore. I had painted the house not long before and I didn't want to have to do it again. At least I hadn't painted the ceilings I guess, well I knew they would have to be redone if I did them anyway because of the roof leaking. For that it had paid off to wait.

With all the raccoons gone we did what we could to patch the hole and replaced the tarp. There were two holes in the roof, and at the time this one was the biggest and the worst. That summer we had more rain and floods than I had ever remembered seeing in my entire life. I remember standing in the kitchen and watching it rain in the kitchen what seemed like as much as it was raining outside. Every single pan and bucket I owned was sitting somewhere in the kitchen and they seemed to be filling up as fast as I could dump them. It was pointless to even try to catch the water because so much was pouring in from everywhere. All the food in the cupboards had been ruined and I wasn't sure if I should even try to use the stove in case water had gotten into anything electrical. I mopped up what I could after the rain

let up and ended up using every towel
we had to finish drying everything off.
We couldn't use our pellet stove for a
while either. Not until we were sure all
the electrical components had ample
time to dry. Oh what a mess that was,
over and over, and of course that year
was the worst for rain. I still refer that
year as the year of the monsoon season.
Finally after a couple years the roof got
done. Well, kind of, that is a whole
different giant can of worms there. We
could not have had a crew that was any
worse to do our roof. They shot at our
chickens with nail guns, destroyed all
the flower beds by the house, dumped
all the roof debris and nails in our
driveway and yard, and the list goes on
and on of all the things they destroyed
and terrorized. They spent eight days
on a roof that is about fifty feet by fifty
feet, and they didn't even do the damn
porch, we had to do that! They didn't
seal any of the roof vents or flashing, so
after an eight thousand dollar roof job it

still leaked like it had never been done and in more places than it had ever leaked before. We had waterfalls throughout the house. We were livid! We will never hire out a roofing job again, not after that experience. They ruined so much of our property and did things I had never dreamed anyone would think to do. I could probably write a book about that horrific experience alone.

The first year Joseph and I had spent together was quite eventful. We can look back at much of it now and laugh. We laughed then too, but not as much as we do now.

Chapter 3
How to Raise Chickens

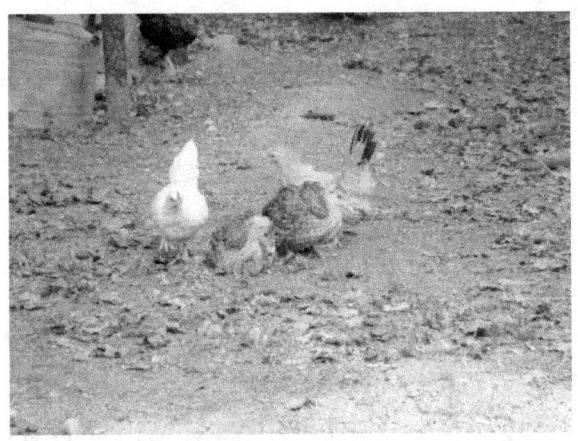

{Here are two mini chickens and two baby turkeys.}

Raising chickens is both an easy and a difficult thing to do. The benefits will always outweigh any negatives as far as I am concerned though. I am no expert on this subject, and we have never stopped learning from daily life around our little farm. So far, most everything we have learned from and have done has worked quite well for us. Everything I will say is my opinion and our opinion on the best way to raise chickens.

Getting baby chicks is easy. They come out in spring around Easter. You can find them at any farm supply store, feed elevators, and they can be ordered from catalogs. Usually a dollar or two a chick depending on the type of chickens you pick out and the area you live in.

Before you get chicks you need to plan for their new home. There are several important things to remember when planning on starting a chicken coop. Another thought, which I seen for the first time not very long ago around the town where we live, is a readymade chicken coop. Just load it in the truck and off you go. I myself thought the coop was fairly small, but I guess most people wouldn't have as many chickens as we do. I would imagine if you have the money that would be a great place to start.

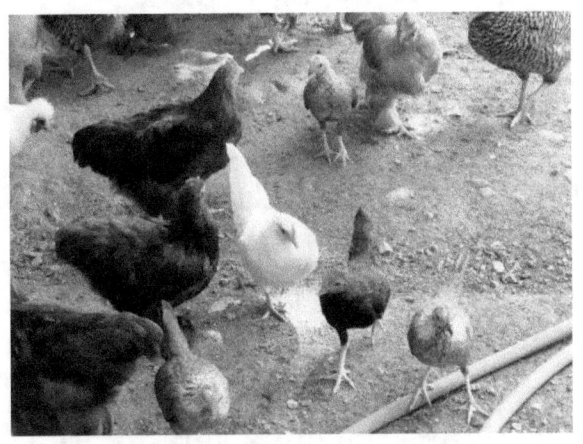

In our case we work a little harder and strive to recycle old or left over building materials from job sites. With the permission of the people in charge of those job sites of course. We would never just help ourselves to anything on anyone else's property without asking first. Around here where we live there is much scrap wood and leftover every-thing to pick from lying around the yard. On more than one occasion all of these scrap piles have proven life savers when emergencies happen and you need something now or at odd hours of the day or night. Then again, when does an emergency ever happen at a convenient time.

Back to the planning for the chicken coop before I get too far off track here. The chicken coop should never be airtight. Having a vented area along the roof edge or in the upper half is an essential part of a chicken coop. Without this vented area to allow air circulation the ammonia smell from the chickens waste can become over whelming. You wouldn't want to gas your chickens or yourself when you venture in the coop to check for eggs either. Yes the ventilation is just as important in the winter months as it is in the summer months. In the summer the smell can get really intense when it is very hot or humid. This is why we have the trap door to allow the chickens to come in and out of the coop into an eight foot by about fifteen foot fenced in area. Give or take a little because I haven't measured it.

If you are going to have a fenced in area for the chickens to go outside without them running all over the yard, make sure you attach a piece of fencing as a roof. If you don't, any critter can and will climb the fence to get to the chickens and you'll wake up to a chicken coop that is empty or full of dead chickens. A roof on the outside pen is also good to keep the chicken hawks or owls from swooping in and killing the chickens as well. There is no way to keep the chickens safe without a roof on any fenced in area.

The floor of the chicken coop should be insulated from the ground. There is a gap of about four or five inches under our coop from where the floor is and where the bottom of the pallet like crate sits on the ground. There is straw packed in this area to keep the floor of the coop warmer in the winter. That was another benefit we found in recycling the old crate, it left room for a good amount of insulation under the floor.

Another consideration is a power source to run heat lamps or water warmers depending on how much money you have to spend when setting up your chicken coop. We need a fifty foot extension cord with a splitter to run the two heat lamps we keep in our coop. Our power is run first to two timers, which then run the heat lamps at different intervals during different times of the year. One bulb is clear and the other a UV heat lamp. We bought those clamp on shop lights and have attached them to boards that were specifically placed in two areas of the coop to hold the lights. When I clamped the lights on the boards, I also used screws to secure the lights so that the chickens cannot for any reason be able to knock the lights down into the straw on the floor. The lights are low enough to provide heat to both the chickens and the water container, but far enough up and away from the walls and floor where the straw is to prevent any fires. That is a very important thing to remember when running any power or hot lamps in a coop. There will be straw in the coop and straw is very easily ignited.

Another important reason to have lights and/or an outside pen is to make sure your chickens get at least eight hours of sunlight each day. They need to stay on a schedule with day and night staying consistent in order for them to keep laying eggs. That is why one of ours lights is a UV and the other clear. One provides the rays and heat they need and the other the brightness of light to mimic day time during short winter days. That is also why I use the timers and set them at different times periodically through the seasons changing. In spring and fall the lamps do not need to be run for as many hours a day as when it's the middle of winter. The red UV lamps are okay at night and don't confuse the chickens into thinking the sun has never gone down. You won't want a clear or bright light running all night long. That will stress a chicken and then you'll likely stop getting eggs.

Over the water containers and the heat lamps we built what looks like a shelf with a slope on top of it. This was done because the chickens will try to roost on just about anything they can sit on in there, and if they sit on those lamps they will burn their feet. When you build a sloped cover, the chickens can't stay on it. So when they fly up to roost on, they just slide right back off. This also keeps them from sitting on the top of the water container and messing all over it. That is another thing chickens will do, mess in their water.

When building a chicken coop, think of it as child proofing as you go and you'll probably end up with a very good set up for your chickens. Just think of chickens as a coop full of curious and mobile three year olds. That should cover all of the crazy possibilities of what a chicken can get into or get hurt on.

You'll want to make sure that all of your doors are easily secured and not easily unsecured by any imposing critters in the middle of the night or while your away from home. Any outside pen you decide to have should not be easy to dig under to gain access to the chickens. It doesn't take long for a neighbor's dog or a coyote to dig under a fence after a chicken. There are several ways to accomplish this. You can bury the fence a foot deep or you can line the outside edges with large logs. We have pretty much done both. The fence is partially buried in spots and is lined in other spots with large heavy logs. Another idea that works well is to dig a small trench under the fence edges and fill it with gravel or pea stone. The gravel is harder for animals to dig in because it falls right back down into the hole they are trying to dig. It's not fool proof, but quite helpful in deterring digging.

You'll want to have nests that are at least a few feet off the floor, chickens like the higher nests because they feel safer up there away from ground dwelling predators. Our coop has nests that go from the floor to the ceiling as well as several old milk crates that are screwed to the walls at various heights. Different chickens have chosen different nests as their favorites. Over all most chickens choose the higher nests. You should always keep straw in the nests for them to cozy into when they are ready to lay eggs. Having straw in the nests will also help keep the eggs from getting broken as chickens come in and out of the nest throughout the day to lay their eggs.

As I mentioned before about the readymade chicken coops I seen. While it is an easier way to get started with chickens, one should always consider the long term. How will you maneuver inside the coop in spring with a shovel to clean the coop out? If the coop is elevated and has a grate on the bottom, then how will you keep the chickens warm in the winter? If I were to buy a readymade coop I would likely make some minor adjustments to the design once I got it home.

The walls of our coop, as I mentioned earlier, are constructed with old barn wood about an inch thick and about twelve inches wide. Though the boards are butted up to one another, there are still small air gaps in each seam. Now while air flow is a good thing, too much is not good. We have a five inch gap along two sides of the roof edge at the top of the coop and the trap door at the bottom on one wall. With that we have more than enough ventilation. In the winter months anything more than those areas is too much to keep the coop warm. We ended up with some thin fiberglass home wrap left over from some job site that was being thrown away. It was in a roll and was similar to thick paper to handle. I used a staple gun and lined the inside walls of the chicken coop with this insulating fiberglass "paper".

As it turns out that was just the right mix of what was needed to keep the coop warmer in the winter but still allow enough air flow. Like I said, we didn't have much of the home wrap. When I ran out I used the bags from the wood pellets from our pellet stove. When I laid the bags flat against the wall and stapled them on, they were like a double lining because I didn't cut the bags. That is still the wall insulation today, and it works great at keeping the drafts from the chickens in the winter. In other areas I have used caulk or insulating spray foam. All depends on what needs to be patched and what we have on hand to patch it with. The chickens have eaten all the foam away, but have not bothered any of the caulked areas. A couple times I have had to patch a slightly larger area because a coon or coyote has tried to dig its way into the coop via the wall. If they can find a small whole or create one, they will keep digging and gnawing at it until they make their way into the coop. In a couple areas I have screwed another piece of wood over an area that has been weakened or has a small hole.

There are two ways to raise chickens; keep them in a coop all the time and feed them, or let them roam during the day and hunt for bugs. A free range chicken roaming for bugs is the best way to have a chicken. The food sources are better than any feed you can buy, and with each bug they get both food and water. When chickens roam they drink much less water, eat much less feed, and lay just as many eggs as they would if you kept them caged in. Another bonus to a free range chicken is pest control. Chickens eat mosquitoes and their larvae as well as flies and many other bugs most people don't want around the house anyway. In my opinion free range chickens are healthier and the eggs are better. In the end it's a personal preference on whether or not you want chickens running around the yard.

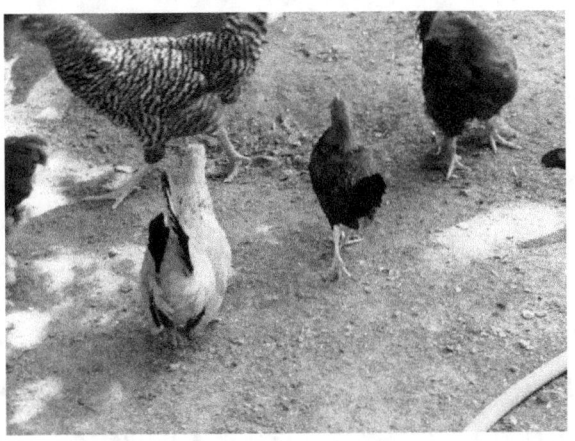

Our coop started out about six feet wide by about eight feet long and probably eight feet tall. We started with about thirty chickens and lost most of them by the end of the first year we had them. Another consideration is if your neighbors have dogs, and whether or not they will keep them on their own property or let them come and eat your chickens instead of their dog food on a daily basis.

The following spring, after we lost almost all of our first chickens, we bought more baby chicks to raise in the house. You can't put new baby chicks in with established full grown chickens because they will kill the baby chicks. We needed an addition to the chicken coop, and added one just a slight bit bigger than what we started with. We once again had come across another large packing crate from a job site where it was going to be thrown away. We built it the same way we did the first section, with more old barn wood. We made another smaller door for this section and once the addition was complete we cut a small hatch door at floor level. The hatch door was cut to be able to separate the coops when we had baby chicks, and open the door to let them travel from one side to the other when the baby chicks were of age to be introduced to the flock we already had. This also gave the chickens enough room that they seem to bicker and fight less.

We did not add an outside pen to this new section because this section would be the one with less air flow to stay even warmer in the winter. This section would also be baby chick proof so that no little ones could escape. This design we had constructed would let the chickens have more than one climate to live in. If the chickens got cold they could go to the new addition to stay warmer, and they did.

When winter is around the corner, there are a couple things you should do for your chickens. One is throw a chunk of lard in the coop when it starts getting cold. You can sometimes get lard from a local meat processor. The lard helps the chickens stay warmer in the winter months much better than just the chicken feed or laying mash will. Chickens will expend more energy when they are cold just like we do. Another thing to not do is clean out your chicken coop in the fall; you should only do that in spring. The manure will emit heat and act as a better insulator from the cold coming up through the floor. When a chicken's feet get cold they won't lay eggs. Only happy chickens will lay eggs.

For the roof on the new addition we used an old piece of thin rubber that was large enough to cover the new roof area, and overlap the original area to keep any rain out. As it turned out, it wasn't completely rain proof. Even though we used caulk and roof tar, it still leaked quite a bit. Someone had given us an old pool shell from a pool they were tearing down and sending to the landfill. We brought the big roll of metal home and it had been sitting out back for a while by then. We had now found a use for it. A new roof for the entire chicken coop. I cut the pieces long enough to span the length of the entire coop and left an overhang on each side. The coop roof is on an angle so I staggered the pieces I cut as you would if you were laying shingles. After the entire roof was re-covered I went back over the screw holes with caulk first and then roof tar to seal any areas that would leak. When I ran out of roof tar I used the silicone caulk to finish off the job. We were in business with a new leak proof roof. Re-roofing over the existing roof proved to be a little sturdier against the wind as well, so the new roof was a double bonus. Even better than anything else, it didn't cost us a dime! I also felt really good about recycling, our new roof was a better place for that pool shell than a landfill.

If you begin to see egg shells that are soft, you should feed the chickens crushed oyster shells, which most laying mash should contain. You can feed your chickens table scraps or old food you've cleaned out from your refrigerator as well. Chickens will eat anything from cake to meat. We keep a bucket hanging in the kitchen and empty it for the chickens when it's ready to be dumped out. If you have chickens, you'll never have a reason to waste any food and it will cut down on the amount of feed you'll have to buy. Chickens see it as a treat as well, so everyone wins. When they see a scrap bowl they'll come running from everywhere.

It is also a good idea to have a good watch dog outside or a live trap so no wild critters can try to get in the chicken coop at night. If a dog is raised around chickens and you introduce the dog to baby chicks when you get them, the dog should protect the chickens and bark when anything comes snooping around your chicken coop. We have a beagle and a Lab/Rottweiler mix. The Lab/Rottweiler is our outside dog and the beagle stays inside. We have a lot of coyotes where we are and leaving a small dog outside is not the best of ideas. Both dogs watch over and protect the chickens simply because we introduced them to the chicks when we brought them home. Or at least I believe that is why they do it. Dogs are very smart for the most part and will quickly learn what they are to protect and warn you about with little guidance from you in that respect from what I have seen. I have noticed that dogs tend to want to please their masters, and when they notice you care for something, I believe they pick up on that.

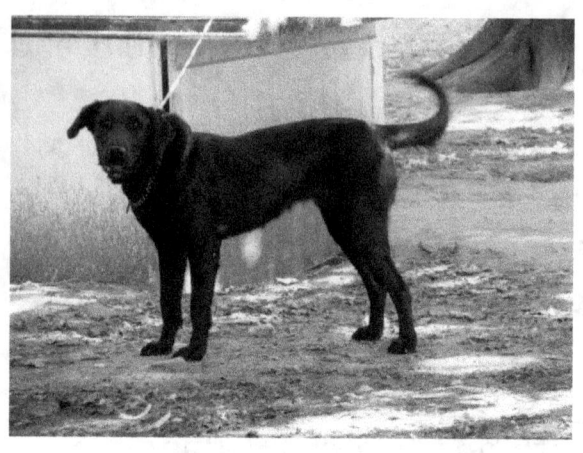

Sometimes we turn the dogs loose to go after any chickens we think may still be out when it's time to close up the chicken coop. Our dogs have never hurt one of our chickens. When I let them loose I tell them to round up the chickens, and they run around in the woods sniffing out where any strays may have gone to hide. When they are on the trail of a chicken I start yelling for them to pin it down for me. They do, they will use their paws to hold the chicken for me until I can run over to pick it up and carry it to the chicken coop. Sometimes we have to do this when a chicken accidentally escapes while we are feeding or checking for eggs. Especially during winter months or when we are getting ready to leave and the chickens aren't going to be let out that day. The dogs are great at tracking, finding, and catching the chickens. When they pin down a chicken for me they are usually holding them by the wings, and have yet to hurt one.

Once all of the initial construction of the coop is finished and your baby chicks have found their new home it will take about six to eight months or so to begin seeing any eggs. That's when the chickens are of mating age and the best time to remove too many roosters from the flock. You should have a minimum number of chickens for each rooster you plan to keep. On average you should have at least twelve or more chickens per rooster. If you don't follow that rule of thumb, the rooster will literally mate the chickens to death. All a rooster will do is keep jumping on the hens he has claimed as his own, and if he doesn't have enough chickens he will over work the ones he has and they will die. That is how people find bloody eggs and unexplainable dead chickens. Having a rooster in your hen house is a good thing, and I've heard it said that the eggs have more vitamin content when a rooster is housed with them. The only time having a rooster will become a problem is if you have to few chickens to support his appetite during their mating seasons. If you find that you have a bloody egg and you know you have an adequate number of chickens for your rooster, then you may want to look elsewhere for the cause. It could be that a cat, dog, or coyote tried to catch or kill one of your chickens. When chickens get scared, they simply won't lay an egg. When a chicken has been physically traumatized or hurt you will see bloody eggs. If that is the case you may want to keep a closer eye on your flock for a while until you figure out what is causing the upset before you start losing your chickens to a roaming critter or a predatory bird.

If you plan to keep a rooster with your chickens, you may not have to struggle with introducing new young chicks should you decide you want more chickens for any reason. Letting the chickens sit on their eggs in spring or fall is the best way to add chickens to your flock. You'll need to know which eggs you should gather every day and which ones to leave under a chicken who is sitting. Use a permanent black magic marker and mark all the eggs under a sitting chicken every day. The chicken won't be very happy about you touching her eggs, but if you're quick it won't be that bad. A chicken will most likely have new eggs under her each day; if not hers then other chickens as well, so always check. If you don't see baby chicks in twenty-one days then the eggs may not have been fertilized and they may not be good. You can get rid of the eggs at day twenty-two if they have not hatched. From what I have seen and been told, if an egg does not hatch on day twenty-one, then it was not a viable egg. Any chicks that we have had hatch one or two days after the twenty-one day mark have never survived.

If the babies begin to hatch, a chicken will only continue to sit for about a week or so. At that point she'll take the babies out of the nest to begin teaching them how to hunt for food. When our chickens have chicks I will take a tiny bowl of water to her nest every day so she can stay in the nest as long as she likes and the babies can get big enough to jump out before they take the first leap. I will also put a hand full of chicken scratch in the nest as well. But I do so discretely, or the other chickens will try to get in the nest to get the food and may hurt the baby chicks or break the eggs to soon and kill the ones that haven't hatched yet. The hen will protect them, but she'll likely have to leave her eggs to do so. I try not to start hen fights, and so I sneak a little handful of food without the others seeing or I will abort the mission entirely until later when I can go un-noticed.

The best part of allowing your chickens to add numbers to your flock on their own is there's no fear of other chickens killing the babies when you try to introduce new chicks to the flock. The hen will protect her young from any bothersome members of your flock and the chickens will accept the new young as part of the flock as they get bigger without much incident. From what I have seen, the first chicken to pick on a hens' baby chick will get its' rear end handed to it by the Mama. That usually only happens a couple times before the others decide they aren't interested in messing with her.

The biggest expense we've expended so far on raising chickens is buying the chicks and the feed. For the most part we have built and patched the coop from recycled materials. In the summer months our chickens are free to roam and hunt for their own food. The feed bill in the summer is quite low. Most times we only have to throw out a few handfuls of cracked corn in the evening. We don't even really have to do that, but we do anyway just in case someone didn't find enough bugs that day. This has cut costs dramatically as compared to raising chickens any other way.

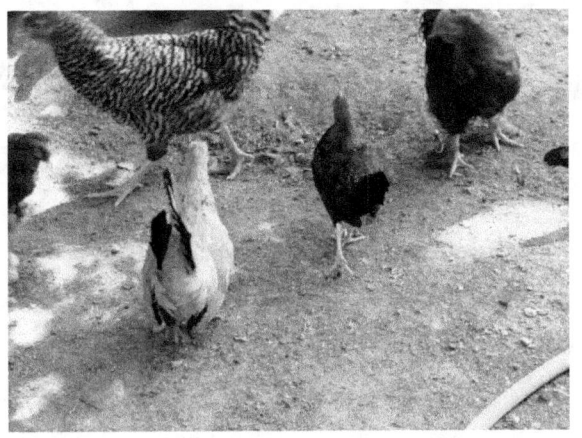

Chapter 4
Why We Raise Chickens

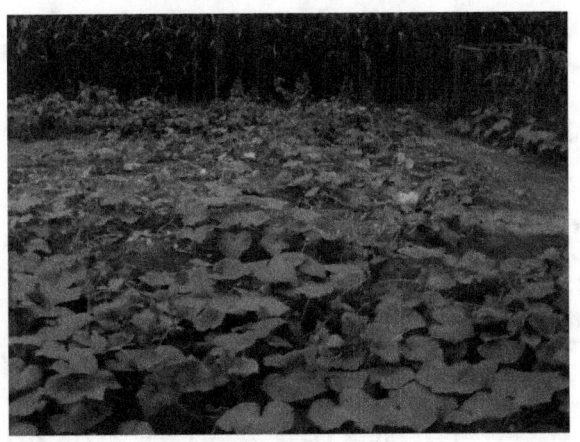

{This is a view of a portion of our garden.}

Joseph and I both grew up with a yard full of chickens. Our parents both had small farms that helped keep the family fed with good, pure healthy food. We both worked on our small family farms. Working on a family farm is a good way to learn responsibility and the meaning and benefits of hard work. We didn't realize it then, but all the work we did as kids made us stronger and more resistant to germs. Eating farm fresh anything made us even healthier and stronger yet. Learning the value of life and the purposes of livestock was an important learning experience for both of us.

Joseph and I were much the same when we left our nests as kids. We stopped eating the things we had eaten when we lived on the farm. The first trip to the grocery store after getting our own place was a rude awakening to just what it was we had grown up with, and how much we were missing the real food we used to eat. As much as we were all in hurry to leave home; when we actually did, we wanted to go back. Even if it was just for a package of home grown meat or a dozen farm fresh eggs. I don't care how much money you have, you cannot buy from any store what can be raised on a small family farm.

There are too many laws which require shots and medications and who knows what else. Everything must be treated in some way before it can be marketed and sold to the public for liability reasons. No matter what, you cannot buy anything that is truly all natural from any standard grocery store or specialty store, you have to know someone you can get it from.

The eggs from the grocery store were a strange pale yellow color, they all had white shells, and they seemed to have no taste at all. I rarely ever bought eggs unless I couldn't find a sign on the side of the road that said farm fresh brown eggs for sale.

When Joseph and I started dating, we realized how much we had in common. Once we moved in together and got married we started our own little small time farming adventures. The chickens have brought us many benefits.

Our yard has fewer mosquito's now, and where we live they are bad. We have several swamps on our property and most of the property is in its natural state. What we refer to it as our own little piece of heaven. We don't disturb much of the wooded areas, which makes up about ninety percent of the seventy acres that we live on. You can only imagine the bugs and spiders that live in our yard. Having chickens has helped in keeping a great many creepy crawlies away from the house and out of the yard.

Another way to view a free range chicken is like a mobile fertilizer. Manure is some of the best fertilizer you can use. As our chickens wander through the yard as mobile pest control units, they also leave fertilizer behind as they eat. I heard people say that manure from chickens has to be aged, or that it isn't useful among other things. Though we haven't directly used it in the garden, it hasn't created any issues anywhere else. We had about one hundred and twenty-five chickens this past spring and given that amount of chickens one may think how dirty our yard must be. Yes, there is the occasional dropping or two that has landed on a brick walkway around the house or in the driveway. It dries quickly and is easily washed away when it rains, or swept away with a broom. With as many chickens as we have that has never been a problem.

I am always running around barefooted in the summer, and believe it or not, I cannot recall ever stepping in chicken droppings at any time I have been walking around the yard. Chicken manure quickly disappears and has never been anything we have had to clean up from anywhere except the chicken coop in spring.

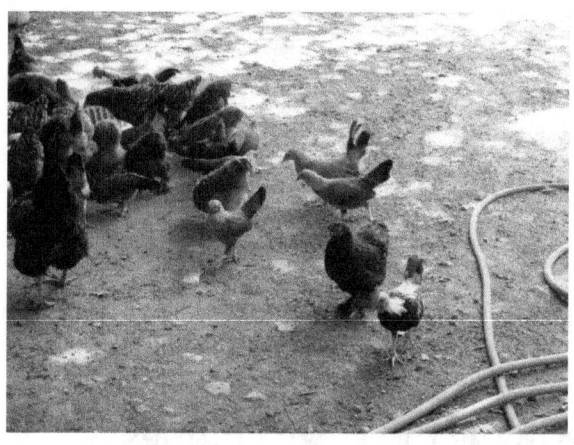

My only complaint about our chickens is that they love mulch. We have elaborate flower beds all over our yard, and the chickens really seem to love to head straight for the flowers and the mulch. This spring the chickens broke three or four flowers off at the base by scratching around the base of the plant in the mulch looking for bugs and seeds that had fallen. While I like the fact they are eating the bugs around the house, we can't afford to keep replacing the mulch. Mulch is way too expensive for that. We only let the chickens out when we can keep an eye on them and shoo them away from the flowers. Here again, we have good cardio when we have chickens. Usually a "shoo, shoo, shoo" will run them off, but for the determined ones they will be back before long. Chickens know where there is food and are stubborn about getting to it. If you have flowers that you don't want chickens to get into you may have to get creative on how to keep them out if you plan have free range chickens.

I tried the little decorative fencing you poke in the ground to keep them out, but that does not work. I am content to shoo them away, and that is a great job for kids to get them off their butts, away from the video games, and give them some exercise as well. It's also a good way for kids to earn extra money if you assign chicken shooing as a chore and give them an allowance.

Another important fact to note is that you cannot hard boil a fresh chicken egg until it has sat in the fridge for at least six to eight weeks. If you try to hard boil it before it sits long enough, then the shell will not peel away from the egg white and you will end up with only a mangled mess and maybe a yoke left after you peel it. That should say something to you about why I won't eat anything but farm fresh eggs. For one, what are they doing to the eggs to make them peel faster than nature intended and/or are the eggs just sitting around that long before you buy them from the store. I don't really care what the answer to that question is, all I know is that eggs from the store aren't natural enough for me, and I don't like how they taste or how they look. We have friends that cannot eat our farm fresh eggs because they don't look like store eggs and it grosses them out to think where they came from. To each his own, we don't really care. All we know is we can't handle store eggs.

In most areas if you have a yard you should be able to have chickens. Unless you live in a city, then you are limited to only hens in some areas, if even that. Where we live we aren't subject to any ordinances prohibiting our raising chickens. If we ever lost our place, I would be the biggest redneck looking hillbilly on the block. You can bet I would have anything and everything I could fit in my yard.

Between chickens and a garden we would not likely have any mowing to do at all. I wouldn't care what anyone thought about it either. Eating real food is more important to me than any manicured lawn that serves no natural purpose and deters anything natural from where I live.

I will show my opinionated side here for a moment. I cannot fathom what dumb ass came up with an ordinance against raising chickens or having a rooster in the city limits (as well as the dog barking thing) due to the noise. Have you ever sat back and listened to what's around you in a city? Loud exhausts on cars and trucks, Harleys that are beyond loud-but perfectly legal, boom boxes from the next block over, road noise, people yelling, and ice cream truck music. All of these things can exist, and be a nuisance all day every day, but you can't have critters that make noise. My dog doesn't bark louder than a Harley and my rooster doesn't crow louder than a Harley. So where is the logic here? How is it logical to only want to hear man made noise?

Forcing people to rescind their freedom of choice to raise organic food. Or to deny people the right to raise small livestock does not seem fair. No, it isn't fair at all. Especially when so many other things are so much more annoying than the sound of something natural. That reasoning just baffles me. I myself could care less about a neighbors barking dog or a rooster crowing, and I can't imagine being selfish enough to complain to any authority about either of those things as well. If that is enough to wake someone up, then maybe they should see a doctor and find out why they can't sleep anyway.

Any good dog will bark if there is a critter or intruder prowling around your home. In my opinion if you can complain about a dog barking, you must not care that there is a reason for that dog barking and you aren't concerned with being warned of such things ahead of time.

In any city I've ever been in the booming speakers, loud exhausts, and squealing tires far outweigh anything else that would wake someone up too early, or bother someone enough to complain. Over all of the noise you can't hear the damn birds chirp in the morning. Birds first thing in the morning aren't really much louder than a rooster anyway. Should they outlaw birds in city limits too? That is just how dumb a law like that sounds to a person like me.

Okay enough about that because I could rant on forever about the ass backwards way people view things in today's society. I wish that more people would realize the benefits of getting back to basics and the importance of revitalizing our farming communities. We need our farms and farmers, and we all need a wakeup call on just how much healthier real food is for our bodies and minds. It's well worth a little noise.

I also hope that if you are able to where you live, that you venture into raising your own chickens and enjoying the goodness in the farm fresh eggs and the fresh chicken should you decide to decrease the size of your flock for any reason. Enjoy the feathers that can be used for crafts when the chickens lose them. Once you get through setting up the chicken coop, for the most part, chickens are low maintenance with the exception of feed and cleaning the coop. That will only need to be done about once a year, and that too will depend on how many chickens you have.

If you handle the baby chicks often when you first get them, your chickens will be tame and friendly. They can, at times, be hours of free entertainment. At any rate, you now know why we feel the way we do about raising our own chickens.

Chapter 5
Chicken Stories

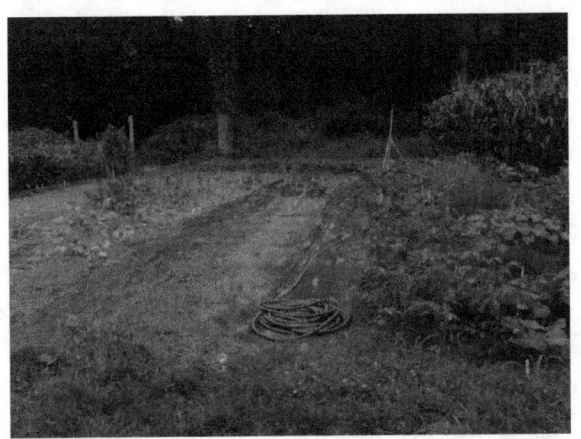

{This is a view of a portion of the garden.}

When we first got chickens I was so excited. Finally, after so many years we would be able to have our own farm fresh eggs again. I had been missing those for way too long, and so had Joseph. When I was young and lived on our small family farm, I treated each and every one of our chickens as pets. I was young and being a farmer's daughter I didn't get out much until I was older. I spent the majority of my time with our animals or working and playing on the farm.

I would spend hours training a chicken or a rooster to do one thing or another. No matter what they did, or didn't learn, they were all always tame because of the amount of time I spent handling them and playing with them. That was the same thing that I wanted for our new chickens when we decided to raise them. I guess somehow I wanted to relive parts of my childhood through these new things that Joseph and I were venturing into as a team. Some of my fondest memories were of times on our family farm growing up. I was ready to make more of those fond memories with my new love.

There is one time that stands out in my mind from my childhood that is really funny to me. My step Dad had gone to town one spring and brought home one hundred baby chicks. I think he ordered them ahead of time, but I'm not sure. There were a couple chicks in the batch that had deformed feet and they didn't look very healthy. I adopted one of the crippled chicks, as I always did. This chick was my new best friend, along with the many others, but this one was different. The poor thing looked pitiful and deformed. We had a four wheeler on our farm and I rode around on it quite a lot. This chick became my new sidekick to ride around with. I named the chick Nibbles. As Nibbles got older, the deformed feet hadn't gotten any better. Nibbles could walk around and hunt for food just fine, but just never was quite right. When Nibbles was on the four wheeler with me it didn't matter how far I went, or how fast I went. Nibbles was completely content to sit in my lap and take in the scenery. There was not a single time Nibbles ever jumped off or even tried to get up from my lap. If I was sitting in the yard, Nibbles would be happy to just sit with me in my lap.

Nibbles got that name because any time I would hold her up to my face and say "give me kisses", she would. She would put the side of her head on my cheek, as if she were giving a hug, and the side of her beak would gently nibble on my cheek. Hence, she became Nibbles, the chicken who gave kisses. One day Nibbles and I were sitting in the yard together and my step Dad came walking up. He had been in the barn feeding the animals, and looking at the now several month old chickens he had brought home. I remember him asking something about wanting to know just how attached to Nibbles I was. I of course had to show him yet again how cool it was that Nibbles would give me kisses whenever I asked. He went on to explain that he was looking at the chickens we had and how he wasn't sure how many he wanted to keep. He was getting ready to get rid of the extra roosters and any chickens that weren't worth feeding because they weren't healthy enough to keep. What he was trying to say to me was that we had several chickens that weren't worth feeding because they wouldn't be productive, and Nibbles was the worst of them all. It doesn't make sense to feed a bunch of farm animals that aren't laying eggs or that you wouldn't want to eat. I knew how many animals we had and that it wasn't cheap to feed them. I also knew that each year he killed the extra roosters and sometimes a chicken or two for the freezer.

Even funnier than this entire conversation we had, which was actually quite short, was the look on his face when I stopped him from explaining his thoughts. I just looked at him and told him that if he wanted to kill Nibbles to go for it. That I knew why he wanted to get rid of the chickens he was going to get rid of, and that I understood. In his amazement he walked away speechless and we were finished with our conversation. I don't think he quite expected me to say what I said or the way I had said it. Farm life is what it is. Some animals stay and some animals go. He warned me of that in the very beginning of our venturing into the farm life, and I fully understood.

You will probably hear (read) me say over and over that planning for everything is the best policy. Here is yet another example of why that can be so important. I went out while Joseph was at work at bought our first probably twenty chickens or so I guess. By the time he got home I had a light clamped to the box and there was a box in the living room that was full of cute little fuzzy chirps.

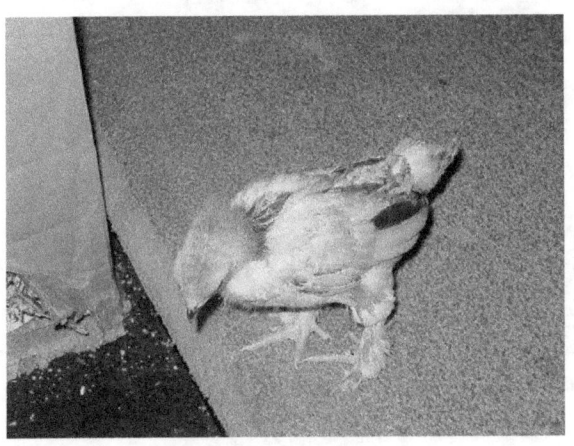

We held the baby chicks and played with them for a long time and we were so excited over our very own first brood of chicks we were to raise together. That was all fine and dandy while it was daylight. But one thing to take note of is chicks don't shut up at night when you have a light on them to keep them warm, just the same as they don't stop chirping during the day. Chicks need the lights to keep them warm for about the first eight weeks, so someone is always running off at the beak.

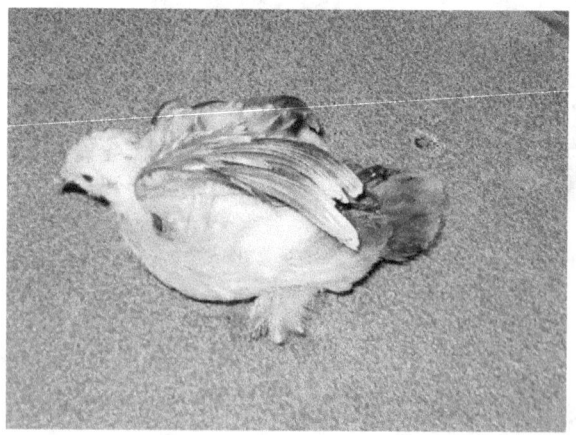

The first couple days were fine because they were still new and cute as little buttons. Like baby chicks always are. Then each day they grow it seems as though their little voice boxes grow as well. Needless to say, Joseph was not very happy that these little fuzz balls were staying in our bedroom. Another thing that wears off after the first week is the box staying clean. It is a very short time after you bring baby chicks home that you end up having to clean the box up to three or four times a day. As the chicks get bigger, the poop gets bigger too. And oh so does the smell. When I bought the water containers and the feed containers, I thought they would help. The water containers would be better than the bowl and would stop the chicks from spilling the water every five minutes. Maybe then I wouldn't have to clean the box every five minutes. Or so I thought. It seems that baby chicks can make just about as big a mess by running through the water. With a proper water container, there is only a small edge of water in a ring around the bottom. One would assume that running through that would not be possible. Well, it was not only possible; it was like the chicks were having a party with a slip and slide in that box. I could say it was hilarious to watch if it wasn't so much darn work to keep cleaning that box so they would have a dry place to nestle in when they napped. That being the case the chicks didn't stay in the bedroom long. They needed to be closer to the sink and the stack of newspapers I was in constant need of. Not to mention the garbage can. Even though I was constantly cleaning that box and I dusted every couple days, at that time you'd have never know it to look at our house.

We had to keep the baby chicks in the house until they were big enough to not escape the chicken coop fencing and until they were big enough to not need a light. I can't remember now exactly how long we kept the chicks in the house, but I know it was well over a month. By the time the chicks were ready to go outside our house looked like a scene from a horror movie. There was so much stinky dust and cobwebs on everything, more than you could imagine could collect in that amount of time. Each time I would wipe something off with a rag I would have to dunk that rag in my bucket. Each time I dunked the rag in the bucket twice, I had to clean out the bucket. That is apparently why chicken coops are so dusty, because chickens emit an excessive amount of dander, or whatever you want to call it. I had to spring clean the whole house from top to bottom all over again. After that I made sure to find all the scrap wood I could possibly find and I built a brooder for the next year. There was no way I was keeping anymore baby chicks in the house for more than a week from then on. It was just too messy.

After the chickens went out to their new coop they seemed quite happy in their new home. A floor and nests full of fresh straw and cute little feeders and waterers waiting for them. They were so tame that they would run up to you and let you pick them up and hold them. As they got older they stayed that way. They would go out and hunt for food during the day and when one of us was around we could pick them up or hand feed them, they didn't mind. We didn't have any roosters with our first bunch of chickens, which was funny because as it turned out there was one hen who sort of led the flock. The rest of the chickens would follow this one hen anywhere she went and it seemed as if they took their directions and/or scolding from her. She was big and white and each and every day she would lay a double yolk egg; without fail. She never laid a regular egg, not once, only double yolks. She was the coolest chicken we have ever owned; even still today I wish we still had that chicken. Compliments of our neighbor's dog we didn't have her for long. I was so furious when I followed the trail of feathers back to the neighbors house that I had to come back home before I confronted anyone. I was barely able contain my anger. We had already asked more than once for them to keep the dogs on their property because they were eating and terrorizing our chickens.

We still have only two chickens left from our original brood of chickens. They are the only smart chickens we have ever had except for about a dozen leftovers at the farmers supply place that were late comers. They were the only chicks in the store the day I stopped in to pick something up. This was the third year we were raising chickens and I had already bought a few more chicks from the farm supply stores. I had gone back to get something, maybe it was feed, I don't remember now. I walked past where they had kept the baby chicks, and there was one little tiny box in the middle of a large cleared area in the floor. I am naturally curious so I had to go look. It was more baby chicks. They were like little cotton balls with feet I swear! There was no price on the box or anything, so I went and asked someone. The guy told me how much they were, which I think was a little over a dollar and a half each. Being poor sucks because there were twelve chicks left and I only had the money to buy ten or eleven, and I just had to have them. The guy was nice enough to give me the chick or two that I could not afford because they just wanted rid of them, and luckily he didn't want to separate them. I came home completely broke but with twelve more baby chicks. Which still ended up in the darn house. We won't go there again. At least I clean all the time, that's all I can say.

Not long after we got them we realized they were different from regular chickens. Regular chickens have three toes and these chickens had five toes. They also had feathers on their feet and they were a medium size chicken with puffy feathers on their heads. They were (are) so cute! Out of those chickens we ended up with a rooster. These chickens, we found out later, were Silkies. Fitting name because their feathers are kind of silky looking and silky feeling. These chickens turned out to be as smart, and smarter than the chickens we had raised in our first year. The rooster would watch over the flock and would not go in the coop until all of his chickens were in the coop for the evening. This rooster would not eat or drink until his hens had both eaten and had water. The second or third winter we had him, we found him dead in the chicken coop. We never did figure out what happened to him or why he died. All I know is I was so sad when we lost him. He was the best rooster we have ever had, and will likely ever have.

Since then we have bought quite a few chickens and had several roosters. I remember how our chickens acted when I was a kid and so does Joseph. Neither one of us can remember a time when a chicken didn't go back to its coop to roost for the evening. Just the same as we can never remember chickens that would not hunt for food, but be content to sit and starve if you don't feed them. These last couple years we have ended up with some of the dumbest chickens on the planet. Some were engineered to be stupid and we will never ever buy another genetically modified chicken ever again. They are sad, abnormal, and they die slow so you have to shoot them if you don't use that steroid filled food for them to grow to weight in like four weeks. They are just all around pitiful! I'm not going there because I won't quit bitching. Back to the subject of the so called "normal" idiot chickens. Animals are born with instincts on how to survive, when you take a wild animal, or even a domesticated livestock animal from its mother when it's young, it still ends up with certain programming from its DNA. Unless you buy most of the chickens they are selling today. I have never in my life seen so many stupid chickens as I have seen in the past three years. I am starting to wonder if all of these chickens that are being hatched and sold have any natural instincts left at all.

Lately we have been getting chickens that don't know how to, and don't want to hunt for bugs. Chickens that won't go back to the roost at night and end up disappearing. And more and more chickens that are eating the eggs they are laying. Are they inbred or something? Or have too many chickens just been sitting in a little cube for too many years and lost all survival instincts? Now I can understand one stupid batch of chickens, but all of them for over three years in a row now? That is starting to look like a bad pattern. The new chickens don't want to sit on the eggs and hatch babies; even after they are well old enough and should be able to. If they hatch babies they don't know how to care for them, and they tend to abandon them and then the babies die. They also don't protect their young as they should. It's like they have no mothering instincts at all. They are beginning to remind me of today's society. (My saying that shouldn't piss you off unless you're one of the guilty ones). I am getting somewhat discouraged at trying to get our chickens to add to the flock on their own, and have decided to look for a farmer that is selling chicks that have been hatched from their own free range chickens. The quality of everything else seems to be falling off in a hurry.

As long as you have enough hens for them, having roosters can be funny. You never know what they'll do next. The last two good roosters we had (and still have) started a big ruckus one day. I could hear all sorts of squawking from the hens and went to check what all the noise was about. There were two roosters fighting and there were several hens standing around watching them fight. The funny part about this is the one rooster is an average size rooster and quite a bit bigger than the hens. An average size rooster isn't small. The other rooster is a bantam rooster, or as

I call them; mini's. Bantams are only about a quarter the size of a regular rooster, but they have the heart and ego of a full size rooster and then some.

These two roosters were sparring quite aggressively and were literally kicking the shit out of each other. The bigger rooster was white and he was covered in blood. The mini was reddish brown, so I couldn't see the blood on him readily. I knew from my childhood not to break them up until they had come to an agreement on their status in the coop amongst themselves. If I had broken them up at that moment, they would only have started their fight up again later, and sometimes they will fight until one dies. If you are watching them closely you can break them up at the moment one surrenders and then the roosters won't go right back at it again in a little while. The fight between these two went on for over another half hour or more I think. They were both so tired they could barely move or stand. They were completely exhausted.

When I was finally able to step in and separate the two, the smaller rooster had finally laid down first and given up. This surprised me because there for a while I thought he was going to kick the big roosters butt. I put them in different places and watched over them until they regained some of their strength.

Once they were up and feeling better they didn't go back to fighting. It's not easy to know when to get between two roosters, but this wasn't the first time I had to do that. Like I had thought, the two roosters were happy with who they felt had won that battle, and who had remained king of the chicken coop and the hens they each had claimed for their own. They did not commence fighting again after that. They both have found their places and seem to get along okay now. It's been three years since that happened and I have yet to see them fight again. If I had stepped into that fight too early. It would be very likely they would have fought again later that night and one of them likely would have died by the next morning with no-one there to separate them when things go to far.

Chickens, like any livestock, can be demanding when it comes to time. They can tie you down to home because they do need to be fed, watered and let out daily in the summer. You can stock them up on feed and water for a few days if you plan on leaving for a short time. Other than that you would need someone to feed and water them for you if you were to be gone any longer. I don't feel I am missing out on anything by tying myself to our small farm. There have been many times when people we know tell us that we need to go out or take a break from work. We enjoy our work because it benefits us and our livestock. We don't view this as a heavy load to carry. It is a blessing that we tend to and live with on a daily basis. We would much rather be here looking out for our livestock and property rather than being in some bar somewhere wasting money we don't have. With the economy the way it is lately. You take your chances when you leave your home unattended for any length of time.

I enjoy this life and spending time in the woods just as much as Joseph does. I enjoy watching the babies grow when we are lucky enough to have them hatch and be cared for by a mother hen.

It is so heartwarming to watch a good mother hen tend to and teach her young how to fend for themselves and scratch for food. Whatever you do, don't threaten her babies or she'll whoop your hind end. Nothing like a good mother in nature, that's the way all mothers should be. Nurturing, loving, caring, teaching, and disciplining to keep the natural balance and keep her chicks in line so they don't misbehave, get lost, or get hurt. I know many human parents who could benefit from a couple hours of watching how good mothers tend to their young on a farm. Maybe I should start the hens parenting class. If I thought it would do any good, I probably would.

My point is that if we can watch and appreciate the natural order of things around us, it can offer us much insight and ways to improve our own lives. Rather than judging and preaching, many need to just sit back, shut up, and learn something. All while enjoying the scenes we see taking place before us.

Chapter 6
How to Grow A Garden

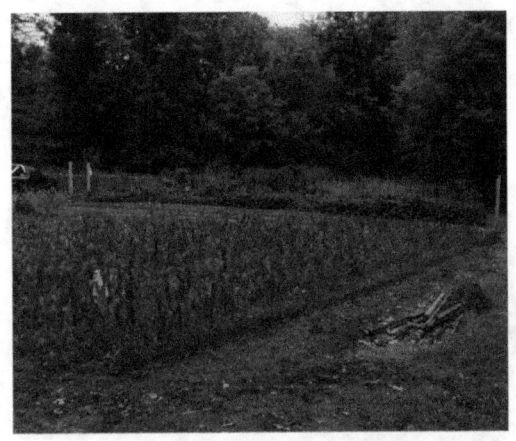

{This is a view from the back of the garden.}

Growing a garden does involve work, but the rewards are priceless. Some of the steps involved in being successful include some research. We don't know everything, but we haven't failed yet so we must be doing something right.

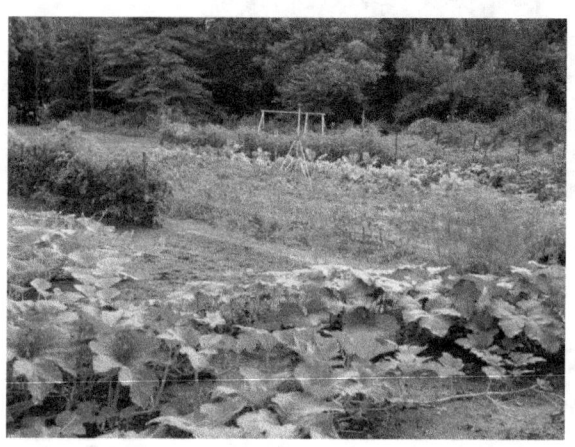

One of the first things to consider is how you plan to turn the soil. You will most likely need a tiller. Depending on your strength and financial resources you may want a tractor with an attachment or a smaller tiller you walk behind to run. There are so many to choose from, but ultimately that will be your preference and what you can afford. I have a cousin who uses her horses to plow her garden. We have a walk behind tiller because we can't afford the tractor and the attachment, but good hard work is the backbone of staying healthy, active, and living a longer life where we come from. If I could afford to feed and keep a horse, I would probably do things just like my cousin does, with a horse.

You need to pick a garden spot that has adequate morning, mid-day and evening sun. Good sunlight is essential to a healthy and productive garden.

When you turn the soil for the first time you may want to spray it with round up to kill any grass or weeds a couple three days before you till. Before you till the first time I would suggest you sprinkle some lime down if you have hard soil and till a second time in a week or two. Whether you need lime or not you will still want to till it again if this is the first time you are using this spot for a garden. You may even need a third tilling for a new garden area. This should kill any weeds and grass that would otherwise be persistent in growing back. We try to till our garden as soon as the ground has thawed enough in spring to allow for tilling. Every area is different so you'll have to look that one up to match where you are.

While tilling we pick out any rocks as we go to try to keep from damaging the tiller. Joseph also demands that anything green gets removed from the garden. The weeds or grass can stay as green manure as long as they aren't at a point where they are ready to drop seeds. Leaving any plant material and using lime to speed the decomposition helps feed your garden necessary nutrients in a natural manner. If they are dropping seeds you'll definitely want to get them out of your garden spot. It is good to have trees close to your garden, but too close will raise the acidity in your garden and you will need to lime it often to counter the acidic effects of the trees and leaves.

Another benefit to having trees around is they are what is known as a shelter belt which allows for utilizing the natural habitat around your garden to help control pests in your garden. Birds like to sit in trees and watch for prey. There will be prey in your garden doing damage to your plants. With natural habitat around your garden, you as well as the wildlife it supports will win.

Some people will use Preen right after they till their garden when they have allowed two weeks prior to planting their seeds. I have been told we should do this, but we haven't managed to get it done yet. I know people who have and they have said it has worked very well for them. If you use Preen two weeks before you plant your garden seeds, it will kill anything that begins to grow through it. Any weed that was still able to grow will sprout and the Preen will kill it. After two weeks it will no longer have this effect and your garden seeds will grow without the weeds following close behind them. If you don't kill all the weeds they will grow faster than your garden plants and will choke out your seedlings. You'll end up having to get rid of the weeds and replanting many of your seeds if you don't keep up on weeding or spraying. Before that happens you will need to pull the weeds by hand or spray carefully for the weeds without accidentally getting overspray on your young plants. You can also purchase plants that have already been started in a green house and transplant them into your garden if you choose. That makes it easier to distinguish the weeds from the plants. Using the Preen prior to transplanting won't affect your purchased plants. Preen will only kill things that grow through it. Transplanting is not the same as growing up through the soil, so it will be fine to transplant before the two week mark with the Preen.

It is also wise to purchase an inexpensive soil testing kit from your local hardware store. Many different stores carry these kits, but we try to spend our money with our long standing local businesses whenever we can. You can get them for around five dollars and up. Depending on how elaborate of a kit you choose to purchase. This will help you decide if you need to add lime to your garden to reduce acidity or if you are missing any trace minerals that would require certain fertilizers to balance. Many times when you frequent your local smaller businesses, they have knowledge-able people who have been working there for years. People who are capable of giving you good advice on what you need and don't need to properly balance you gardens ph level and mineral contents. One thing you should never do is just start throwing fertilizers down when you don't really need them. That only adds unnecessary fertilizers to an area which can run off and be detrimental to the watershed and effect the environment down river as well as your own area. This can cause long term negative effects in waterways and on the environment as a whole. So being sure of what you need is important, not only for the money you will save, but also for our environmental future.

When you plant, be it from seed or transplanting purchased vegetable plants, it is always a good idea to label what you have planted. Labeling is especially important if your garden is large like ours. It can be easy to forget what should be growing in any given row and it makes it easier to know what you should be pulling out should weeds begin to show up with or before your baby plants. There are many weeds that closely resemble many different garden plants. It can also be a good idea to hold onto any seed packets you have purchased to reference back to the sketches on the backs of them. These sketches will show you what your young garden plants will look like when they should begin to grow. As your plants grow taller you may want to invest in some cages or stakes to help hold up your plants when it rains or if a storm moves through. There are many inexpensive ways to accomplish this, and once you invest in these cages, stakes, or both. You'll be able to use them year after year.

Joseph and I are both bow hunters. Sometimes when you target practice you can bend or lose an arrow. Sometimes we find old bent arrows later and pick them up and bring them back to the house. Many people might just throw them away. We save everything. This year I started using the old and bent arrows as tomato and bell pepper stakes. They worked out great. One more bundle of garbage that we found a use for that did not have to end up in a landfill.

Another consideration when choosing a garden plot is the amount of wildlife you will be trying to keep from eating your garden. Should you have a fence, an electric fence, a scarecrow, or a gun? If you have very many deer, they will jump a fence quite easily. If you have a scarecrow, how long will it remain effective before the wildlife gets used to it and no longer pays it any mind? I have been weeding in the garden more than once and had deer standing on the edge of the garden staring at me and stomping their feet. As if I was in their grocery store or something. I have never bothered with a scarecrow for that reason. The animals around here tend to come quite close to me, so what good would a scarecrow do us? Probably not much.

If you have a fence, can you move it twice a year to till your garden? Where we live, we have every critter known to man, and we can't feasibly put up a fence either. The garden is too big and keeping the grass mowed up to the edge would not work if we had a fence. Weed whipping inside the fence would spray too much debris back in the garden for our liking. Why waste the extra fuel to weep whip? The weeds are bad enough and we sure don't want to add to that problem. We haven't yet figured a way to fence that big of an area. It would need to be easy enough to remove and replace to be able to till. The ideal fence for a garden should be buried. If it were fenced in, then I wouldn't be able to drive around the garden to make it easier to load what I'm picking in the back of my truck. Or in the little wagon depending on how much I am picking on any given day. Yes our garden is just that darn big. It seems every year Joseph finds a way to justify making it another hundred square feet bigger!

Here are several old fashioned critter control techniques we implement. One of the biggest complaints we here from people we know is the damage deer are doing to both vegetable gardens and flower gardens. Our answer to that which works quite well, but nothing is one-hundred percent, is dog hair. Deer see a dog or a coyote as a natural predator right? Right. Leaving the scent of a dog or a human where they are headed to will deter them from venturing into your garden. There is only one problem with this; you need a steady supply of human hair and/or dog hair and the dirtier it is the better. The more of the scent it emits from the object a deer doesn't like is that much more of a deterrent. After it rains a couple times the scent diminishes and the deer begin to invade the garden again.

When I bought my bag less vacuum cleaner I thought I was doing a good thing. I was quite happy cutting down on excess paper waste by not having to purchase vacuum cleaner bags all the time. Not only did I cut down on waste, but we have a dog in the house and I do all the hair cuts in our house which also gets vacuumed up. Not only does hair keep critters away, it also contains nitrogen which is also a fertilizer. Dumping the bucket from the vacuum cleaner in the garden turned out to be great critter control and a natural fertilizer! I would dump it in a line starting around the backside of the garden and continue the line around the garden each time I dumped the bucket. When my line was complete around the garden and if it was still working I could sprinkle it around in the garden as well. It kept the deer and the rabbits out for the most part. The rabbits were much quicker to come back though. I had started a box to keep the vacuum cleaner contents in until I had time to walk it across the road to dump it. That wasn't the best of ideas because I didn't want it in the house, and it would get damp being out on the porch if it rained and sometimes it would mold. I haven't had to do that for a while now, but if you need too and you can do it, it works fairly well.

Another solution to rabbit control is something called blood meal. It is in the fertilizer section at your local hardware store. It is nothing more than dried animal blood. Hence, the name blood meal. This is applied in the same fashion as with the vacuum cleaner bucket. A line around the garden will be effective until it rains and washes it away or into the ground. Blood meal is used to repel rabbits as well as another great fertilizer. It can be somewhat expensive though, especially if your garden is as big as ours. To run a line around our garden we need to buy about fifty pounds of blood meal or more if we want to have a little left to fertilize with. Running a thick line around the garden and then sprinkling it throughout your garden is quite beneficial. It is also natural and poses no threat to the environment.

The ground hogs are the problem child in our neighborhood. I have found nothing that will deter them from the garden, and they are hard to catch in a live trap, even with carrots. They are very smart and leery of everything. My only solution to them is a bullet. Yes, a bullet. If I am to choose between my hard work and food or the ground hog. I think you already gathered who loses that battle.

Let's get back to the growing and nurturing your new garden. If you have tomato plants, you should cover the soil under the plants to prevent any fungus in the soil from killing your plants. I have been told that sprinkling corn meal under tomato plants will kill the fungus in the soil and keep your plants healthier longer. This is one thing I have yet to try. Trying this is harmless to anything in your garden if it doesn't work, so I thought I'd throw it out there. I am not very wealthy and I happen to love corn bread. I have not been able to part with my cornmeal yet, but one of these days when we have some extra money we will try that. Using mulch under tomato plants is another way to keep them healthier, only problem being you should not till mulch into your garden every year due the acidity increasing with the wood. Also some types of mulch will develop fungus quickly and only add to any fungus problem, and maybe even create one. Using newspaper or garden matting under tomato plants is the best way to protect them from any soil fungus. If you already read the newspaper anyway, then it is also kind of a free solution to blocking fungus from the soil. Just find a place to stack the newspapers until garden season arrives, and once you use the newspapers in your garden they can be tilled right in at the end of the year or pulled up, shaken off and recycled or re-used. Of course you should only use the black and white portions of the newspaper for this purpose. You just lay the papers down and spray them with the hose. They do need to be rather thick for this to work though.

Most of the other vegetables we plant are fairly easy to grow, like beans, peas, corn, carrots, etc. I have found that using tomato cages for the green bean plants is better for that purpose than for the tomatoes. The tomatoes always out grow the biggest of tomato cages and snap off at the top anyway. We set two treated four inch by four inch posts on either end of our rows of tomatoes. Then we drilled holes through the center and attached a cable with cable clamps across the row of tomatoes. When the tomatoes get tall enough where they need to be supported I gently tie garden twine loosely around them and tie them to the cable above them. This gives them some stability in the wind and rain, and they aren't as likely to outgrow this type of support system and snap. As the tomato plants get taller, I shorten the garden twine to accommodate the growth. This isn't a perfect solution, but it does work a lot better than the cages do for us. The peas are happy with a scrap piece of fencing, a tomato cage, or any trellis like teepee you provide them with.

For lettuce and cabbage and other greens, Joseph constructed these large cages from scrap would slats and left over scrap fencing. They are huge squares that are almost four foot by four foot by four foot. The top is open as well as the bottom; it is the sides he covered with fencing. When we set these cages over the plants, it is too small for the deer to jump in, and too tall for them to reach down and eat the plants. It seems to keep the ground hogs, rabbits, and other small critters out of the areas we have cages enough to cover. The birds will still fly into the cages to eat the bugs they see. The cages are light enough that I can tilt them over some to reach in and pick what I'm after. This was a brilliant idea that has worked very well; I am hoping we can come up with material enough to make a few more of these cages. Once again this was another great way to recycle scrap material that would have only ended up in a landfill. Yet another way for us to accomplish what we needed to, and without having to come up with money we didn't have to get it done.

When the garden is harvested the corn stalks can be cut and used for decoration around your house, and the extra can be sold for a few extra dollars. You can pick and carve as many of your own pumpkins as you can grow or you can sell any extra for extra money as well. Pumpkins can be fed to chickens after you are finished with them as lanterns on your porch in fall. Deer like them as well.

Any leftover plants that are dying for the season can be left until fall to help prevent soil erosion and tilled in with lime as green manure which will help fertilize your garden naturally. They can also be plucked and composted in spring before your first tilling. Either way we have still seen no waste with gardening. Much can be done naturally saving the cost of many chemicals which can be unnecessary and even damaging to the environment.

If you need to water the garden, using a drip hose that is run along the ground is the best and most effective form of watering your garden. It cuts down on excess water evaporation and keeps you from burning the plants in the sun when they are watered from overhead. It uses the least amount of water to effectively water the plants which also cuts down on the electricity bill if you have well water, or the water bill if you have city water.

Should you live in an apartment, you can also do what I did when I lived in an apartment. You can use your balcony to hold potted garden plants and bring them in the house in the fall if you can. One bit of advice that I learned the hard way; never use blood meal in potted plants of any kind!!! Trust me on this one. I won't give you the nasty details, just don't do it!

If you have been wanting to grow a garden, but just haven't felt ready yet. I would have to believe that I have provided enough information for you to be quite successful at your first attempt. Trial and error can figure out anything that's left to learn. That will hopefully continue your interest in growing a garden every year. Even if it is only a small balcony in an apartment that yields a few fresh veggies. Once you have tasted a garden fresh vegetable, I doubt you would ever want anything that wasn't from a garden after that. If you already have a garden then I hope some of our down home practical critter control will help you in your yearly garden. There will always be more to learn when gardening; it seems we learn something new every year. As with most things, what works well for us may not work for you. We all learn from friends and family, tips about this and that. When it comes down to it, we are all still figuring it out. It doesn't matter how old or experienced we are.

When it comes down to it, having a garden will get you out of the house for some fresh air and some good exercise and give you some of the healthiest food you could ever ask for.

Chapter 7
Why We Grow Our Garden

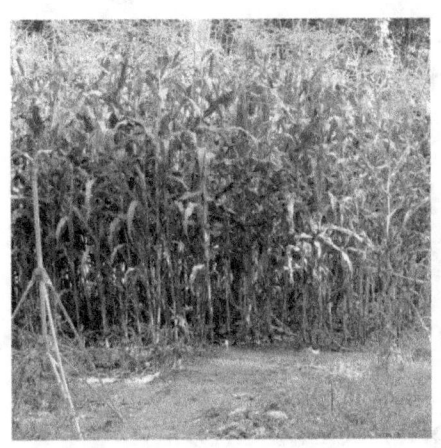

{This is a closer view of the corn.}

When you grow up eating such good natural foods, like those from a garden. It's hard to forget how good those vegetables used to taste when you were younger. Every time I would buy something from the store after I moved out on my own, it never seemed to taste the same. It lacked flavor and was always coated in some thick nasty wax I couldn't seem to wash off. There was also a lingering chemical after taste that reminded me of bug spray. With each year after I left home the produce at the markets only seemed to be getting even worse.

Joseph and I both shared that same experience and neither one of us ever really bought much produce of any kind unless it was from a farmer's market or specialty organic store. I hate to say it, but buying from organic stores is most certainly out of our budget. We have only been able to afford to shop at the worthwhile organic places about twice in the last six years. For a budget like ours that was usually way out of the question. That or we could only afford two or three small things for the whole week. One of the stores we went to seemed to buff and polish their produce just like any other non-organic market would. Why would we pay more for the same thing we we're trying to pay more for to avoid? Even at those organic places, though they were way better than the chain stores, they still weren't as good as home grown. The only alternative left became to grow our own.

When we first started our garden we were as poor as we are now, and we started with an ancient tiller Joseph found on the side of the road that was only fifteen dollars because it needed work. When he first used our new treasure to till the garden Joseph had to hold the cable that ran the drive tines and the handle with one hand and the other hand had a grasp on the other handle. So he essentially tilled the garden with only one hand. Now that is what you call hard work and determination. Making do with what we have to because we are trying to do better for ourselves. The first year of our garden was pretty bad for weeds. We didn't have the money for sprays, and at that time I wouldn't have allowed any to enter the garden anyway. I wanted purity at its best. I have worked my tail off for that cause ever since. I spent most of my time in the garden the first year because I was out of work half the summer. My ten hour days were free, but at least we could benefit from the hard work I put into the garden. At least I could get a tan out of the deal. With me not working at the time, the savings on our grocery bill was much needed. We ended up with plenty of pumpkins to carve and corn stalks to decorate the house with for fall and Halloween. We ended up with plenty of canned goods for the winter and fresh corn on the cob waiting in the freezer for a cold winter day. There is nothing like the taste of good sweet corn in the middle of winter to remind you why you grow a garden.

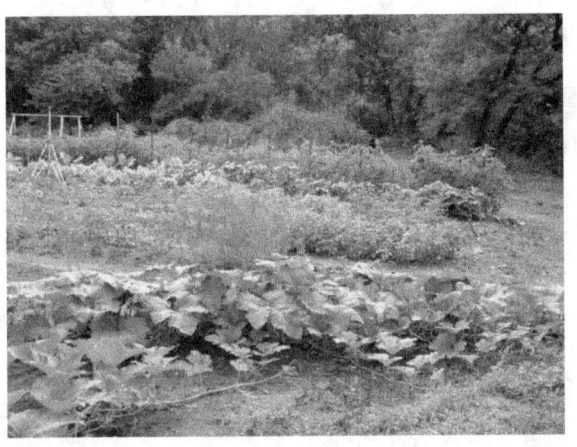

Not only do we grow a garden because it is good exercise. We do many of the things we do because it saves on money and it is so much better for your body when you eat real natural foods. The number one reason(s) is for the actual taste and nutrition you get out of something you grow yourself.

I still remember the first time we picked our first tomato we had grown together. We stalked that tomato for weeks. Checking on it every day and waiting for it to turn red. The mouth watering aroma and the burst of flavor. We couldn't believe we hadn't remembered just how good home grown tomatoes were, and just how horrible what we had been eating from the stores had been. I mean we knew, but the flavor was even better than both of us could remember because it had been so many years since we had a real home grown tomato. To this day we wait, watch and drool over the gardens first tomatoes of the season. Just like kids in a candy store.

Joseph and I had gone shopping one day and we were both craving fresh fruits and vegetables as we were walking around. Obviously if we were craving it, our bodies needed it. We only had about a hundred dollars left over for the rest of the week and we weren't sure if we should spend it. All of that fresh fruit and the fresh vegetables looked so good that we ended up spending almost every dime we had. We got home and dug right in. I started on the grapefruits and he started on the oranges. The grapefruits were okay enough to eat, but were like eating water that had partially evaporated with a skin around it. A grapefruit is supposed to have zip and zing, and be a little sour, but not these grapefruits. From there I tried a plum, another wonderful piece of zippy fruit. I like zippy in case you hadn't already noticed. Nope, not a bit of flavor. I spit it out it tasted so bad. It was like a three day old damp and nasty kitchen sponge in my mouth. Joseph was saying the same thing about the flavorless oranges. We both tried the peaches and the nectarines and we were both absolutely disgusted. Next was the watermelon. Well, need I repeat the same lines over and over? Not a shred of flavor and not very juicy. We sliced the cucumbers hoping for at least one thing we had brought home to have some flavor. I spent about ten minutes with mild soap and a sponge trying to remove that thick nasty wax that was all over this cucumber without much luck. I ended up having to peel it because that wax was so thick. We sliced the cucumber and sprinkled it with a pinch of salt and we both took a big bite. We both spit it out. It tasted like pesticide and no other noticeable flavors other than that. All that money we had spent and we fed every bit of it to the chickens because it was so horrible. It all looked good and was very shiny, but it tasted like shit to put it nicely. We were broke and still hungry at the end of that deal, and it quite frankly pissed me off.

There is one store we go to all the time where we get the best of the store bought fruits and vegetables there are to be had without actually going to the farmer's market. Our famer's market is only one day a week and only in the morning. We never make it in time. Still, there is nothing I have tasted yet that compares to real home grown food except a couple stands in the farmer's market. We managed to make it there only twice and were very pleased with the produce we got from a couple of the old timers who really know how to grow good food. I was even more pleased to have the opportunity to ask the grower himself about the chemicals used to grow the food. I did find a worm or two in one or two things I brought home. That only tells me that when the farmer said he doesn't use chemicals. He wasn't lying to me. I am quite happy to cut that little portion out and enjoy the real flavor of the rest of that natural vegetable.

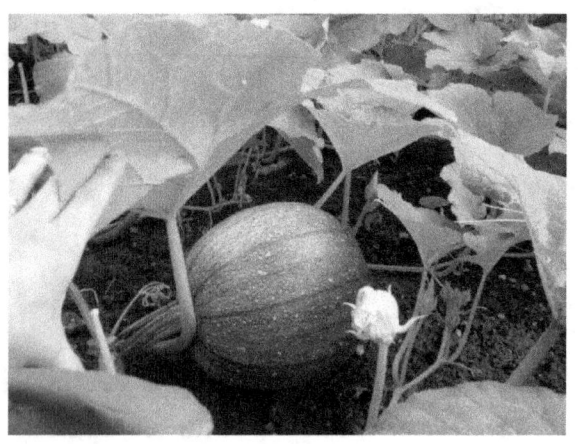

Big business has become so concerned with the bottom line that they have forgotten why the product should be more important. I often wonder if other people buying produce from the grocery stores realize exactly what it is they are missing when they take that nastiness home. I also wonder if we are the only ones to take it home and then gag on it. There is one major chain that is particularly horrific every time. The same store where we spent the last of our money on all that produce that we had to throw away. I wonder if other people actually consume the produce from this store. To us it just doesn't seem possible. Even my dog wouldn't eat it and she loves fresh produce. We can't be the only ones who say we'll never buy it again.

Another fact that many people don't realize with any purchased or processed foods, especially fast foods, is what they are actually eating. When Joseph and I got back to our childhoods and began gardening, we began eating better than we had in years, which goes without saying. Closer to the end of the season we get really busy and sometimes have to run through a drive through or order a pizza because there is no time to slow down and cook. Hell a lot of time it's a luxury to have the time to take a shower around here with as busy as we stay all the time. There is way more to our daily routines than just a garden. Life, work, kids, and a farm gets rather hectic (but worth it no matter what). We began to notice that we would get sick every time we ate fast food. Each pizza would send us fighting over the bathroom for a couple days! We would immediately get stomach aches after we ate or bad stomach cramps. I'll spare you the details on that, I'm sure you know what that means. At first we thought we had a bad batch or something, then it happened every single time we went anywhere. We traded pizza and fast food for restaurant food when we could afford to, and we got sick with each and every restaurant we ate at as well.

Then we began to see a bigger picture. Our bodies had been living off such pure food that the chemicals and additives in all of the processed foods would make us sick each time we ate it. We have found only three restaurants we can go to dinner at, and not end up ill afterwards. Only two fast food places that won't make us sick as well.

Even more interesting is the other things we began to change in our lives and what we noticed with those changes was astounding. I remember when I was in high school, a friend of mine was telling me about this company she had gone to for a job in sales. I think she was peddling some kind of all natural something and had attended a seminar. She began telling me about how bad Teflon coated pans are and how they cause cancer and whatever else she said it causes. She went on to say that the ingredients in deodorant cause Alzheimer's and something else I can't remember. These conversations we had were floating around in my head all of the sudden and I hadn't thought about those times we had talked in over sixteen years.

I remember attending a seminar myself when I was a teenager. In that one seminar I had heard that fluoride was nothing more than a chemical big business was getting rid of by putting it in toothpaste. That fluoride did nothing to actually prevent cavities; fluoride would in fact help cause them and other problems. More over how artificial sweeteners would cause brain damage if you used them all the time. How the artificial sweeteners would rot your teeth from the inside out, instead of the normal outside in tooth decay that regular sugar supposedly causes. I heard about how immunizations were not the smartest decision to make for your kids because they weren't safe. That they could cause autism and a multitude of other debilitating conditions. Many years later, now those shots are actually being linked to autism, retardation, learning disorders and who knows what else that I haven't heard of yet because I hate television for the most part. With an exception of Criminal Minds anyway. Other people are reacting to certain vaccines and they are dying. The funny part about that is (well not funny but stupid), if you tell your doctor you don't want that for yourself or your kids; they get pissy with you ninety percent of the time. Apparently it pisses them off if you value your health and life itself more than any vaccine or what they recommend. I have hardly ever had good experiences with any health care professionals.

In other travels I have learned that plain chocolate wasn't bad for your teeth and was told it's actually good for your teeth. All of the chewy and sticky stuff is what rots kid's teeth out. I've heard that fast food uses additives that cause you to be hungry quicker and make you feel the need to eat more. This is just another underlying ploy they can use to keep you coming back and increasing their bottom lines for them. I've heard that additives in lunch meat were dangerous. I read an article in our local newspaper about a boy who suffered from extremely severe symptoms like migraines and something else. He missed a lot of school and was in misery much of the time. As it turned out, after many doctors and many years later, this child had an allergy to the chemicals injected into processed lunch meats and hot dogs from what I remember. I could go on forever on this subject. Most of it I believe and it appears to have come from what I considered credible sources back then and the same thing now. I highly doubt the lady in that newspaper article would have fabricated the long and in depth story warning other parents of her sons' plight. Though the industries affected by her findings would have you believe that was the case.

When I was a kid, the only kids who were so called ADD were kids who were either born from alcoholic mothers or kids who completely lacked any discipline or boundaries. There weren't three-hundred medications hitting the market every year and I had never heard of Alzheimer's. The medications had been properly tested for extended periods of time before hitting the market. Now you are the lab rat with any and all new medications. If enough people die, they might recall it. Then again, they might not.

Now there is a pill for everything and it seems a disease for each pill. When I was young I remember a lot of seventy years olds were still puffing away on Lucky Strikes or spitting tobacco. Many had never seen a doctor because they were always healthy. They didn't get a cold every season, and neither do I since I stopped eating food that we don't grow. One great big difference between that generation and now is they ate good food that they grew and they worked more than they sat around in front of any TV or game system. There was no such thing as a twelve year old having a heart attack at school while playing sports back then. Life styles and life choices are completely different now, and they are not for the better. I don't care how much technology has improved our lives, nothing can ever replace getting off your butt to do some good old fashioned work and eating healthier as a byproduct of all that work you've done to eat better.

I rarely get sick anymore, even when I'm around kids that are sick. I have a much stronger immune system since I began eating what we grow and what we kill.

Joseph has seen the exact same change in his immune system. We won't take antibiotics unless we absolutely have to because that will stay in your body until you cleanse it out. I guess it causes some people to gain a lot of weight if they don't know how to get rid of it after they have used antibiotics. I use natural methods whenever I reasonably can. Joseph is the same way. I flat refuse to take any new medication of any kind. If it hasn't been on the market for at least twenty years then I want no part of it. I was on a medication at one time that I later found out was causing heart attacks in healthy and active young people and causing internal bleeding. Yeah, let's say we will help your problem and hope you don't die! Screw that. All I have to do now is figure out how to get rid of arthritis and what causes it and I'll be all set. Then again, when your body is craving a certain something you should listen. Your own body will tell you what it needs. As long as you feed it something natural and healthy, it should be happy with you.

Once I quit using whitening toothpaste, my teeth got whiter. My breath didn't smell like a breath mint, but I haven't been handed one yet either. That must be a good sign. I use baking soda now. I stopped using deodorant. I cleaned out my kitchen and got rid of every Teflon coated pan I had. They became dog bowls and some went to the landfill, as much as I hate doing that.

I hadn't worn deodorant in probably a year, and we had been eating at home the entire time because we were tired of getting sick every time we went out to eat. There came a day when we were busy and we went to one of the places we knew we could eat at and not get ill. Keep in mind here that I only shower every other day and I sweat like a hog working outside in the garden, in the house, and around the farm. I had not once smelled of body odor during that time. I guess up until this point I hadn't really noticed or even cared if I did. Like the pigs or chickens care if I stink. An hour after we had gone out to eat, we weren't sick, but I stunk like an old dead carcass in the road. My armpits could've knocked anyone out! I was so grossed out I took a shower. As I continued to sweat the stench returned. The next day I took another shower, and apparently by then my body had excreted all of the toxins or whatever additives were in the food I had consumed the evening before, so the stench did not return.

Now that this had happened, we started paying more attention. We noticed that each time we ate out at the "safe" places, we would still stink beyond belief until our bodies had finally expelled all of the toxins we had consumed with our meal. Though some places we eat at the after affects are way less than others, it still means something about what exactly it is that you are consuming. Finally Joseph stopped wearing deodorant and he too didn't smell of body odor when he would work. He works hard and he always came home stinky before, even with deodorant. Not anymore, as long as we ate at home, neither one of us would smell!

Oh, and his shoes stop smelling bad too. Joseph used to have to use baby powder in his work boots because his feet would stink, and my feet used to stink too being in sweaty work boots all day. Now you could put your nose right in both of our shoes and not smell a thing. If that doesn't tell you something about the crap we consume from so called big business, then nothing will.

I only use cast iron skillets to cook with now and will use my old aluminum pans for baking, but no more of this new fancy stuff anymore. I use wooden spoons and always laugh when someone comes for dinner and they can't believe how good our foods is. I make everything I can from scratch to avoid processed boxed foods from the store. We of course use flour and sugar even though I don't like to because its bleached and treated and who knows what else. But we cannot afford the finer all natural flours and grains so we are stuck with that until we hit the lottery I guess. At any rate, all we do has been enough to make a huge difference. Not just the difference in the grocery bill, but our health as well. On average I spend less than twenty dollars a month on groceries. That is usually for milk or butter. Sometimes

I'll spend a little more if I have to stock up on flour for baking or vinegar for canning or cleaning. Yes, I do occasionally buy a little junk here and there. Joseph does love Velveeta.

It's funny because sometimes people will ask me what kind of perfume I am wearing, and when I am not wearing any and it makes me giggle. I guess when we eat pure food our bodies don't smell all that bad. All I know for sure is we will never, ever be without a garden again.

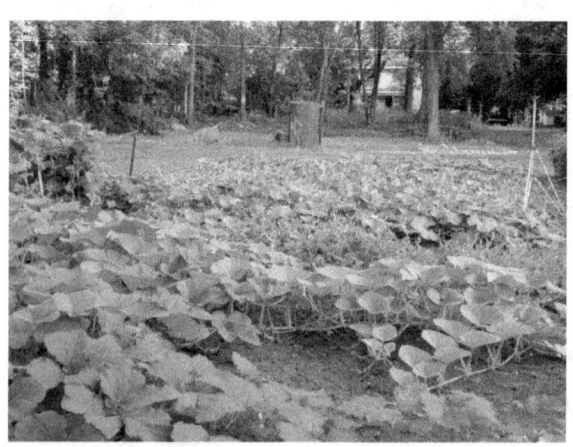

Chapter 8
Garden Stories

{This is a picture of one of our cabbage plants.}

The garden is usually a fairly quiet place if you don't count deer or ground hogs. Here not too long ago I was out pulling weeds in the garden and all in a matter of a half hour it seemed almost chaotic. No, it didn't just seem chaotic, it was!

I was bent over pulling weeds when a chicken started going nuts in the tall weeds directly behind me. She was about fifteen feet behind me I guess. I looked back and all I could see was a chicken that kept flying straight up and down and squalling like it was being tortured. Each time it flew up I could see it and it looked fine. As I was running over there to figure out what the heck was going on I still couldn't see anything. I know the weeds were every bit of four and five feet tall, but they were tall and not very thick, so there was some visibility through them. I ran right in there and still couldn't see anything on the ground under her that would cause her to act like she was. The chicken ran out when I ran in and went across to another section of tall weeds. I stood there for a while watching and listening, but still nothing. I went back to pulling weeds and a few minutes later I stood up to stretch out because my back was getting stiff. As I stood up I caught movement out of the corner of both eyes. One right in front of me and the other halfway across the garden, probably about thirty to forty feet away from where I was standing. The one closest to me is the one I tried to chase. It was a mole. I lost it after cutting it off in the garden after about the seventh time. After that one disappeared I headed for where I last saw the other movement, it was also a mole. It took off across the garden and I chased it as well. I was running everywhere it went and kept cutting it off. That one I eventually killed, but the other one I never did find. Laughing to myself at how eventful the day was turning out to be, I went back to pulling weeds.

I raised up to stretch again, because I had been at pulling weeds for a long time, like all day, and was starting to stiffen up. It was getting to be about five or six o'clock by now. When I looked up I seen another bit of movement in the corn. It was a rabbit headed for the lettuce. Out here rabbits around our house are a nuisance when they get over populated. When their population isn't that high I can use blood meal around the garden to keep them out, also when I can afford blood meal and this wasn't one of those times. Other than that they get shot. Yep, they get shot. I walked over and pulled out my 9 millimeter Sig Sauer pistol and plugged one round in the lettuce thief and I was off to work again pulling weeds. That's when I seen bunny number two. How this one had been in the same row I was in and how I hadn't already noticed that is beyond me. I took a shot at number two and it was a close but no deal shot. This one got away. As I turned from that to go back to weeding I didn't to expect to see anything else after taking a couple shots. I went back to weeding. Go figure, the next time I looked up I saw more movement. Only this movement was completely different from anything I was used to seeing, or had ever seen for that fact.

It was running out of the weeds and toward me in the garden like it was Peppi Le-Pue from Bugs Bunny. I can't say that I ever remember seeing how you spell that name come to think of it. Anyway, it was red with a white belly and was bouncing up and down on all fours at the same time. Whatever it was I had never seen one before and it was neat. I started walking toward it and it was headed toward me. I thought we were going to meet each other for a minute. It changed its direction and headed closer to the edge of the tall weeds and the sat there looking back at me and watching me. I got about fifteen feet from it before it decided to go another few feet and then stop and look back at me again. I was almost to it when it took off into the tall weeds never to be seen again, well at least not yet anyway. When Joseph got home I started going on about all the critters that ran by me while I was weeding in the garden. Then I was asking him if he knew what the last red one with the white belly was. He didn't know, and I thought it must be of the weasel family so I started looking. I got on the internet and typed in weasel and a cute little picture of that same little creature I had seen earlier popped up first thing. Oh how cute they are. After all the years we have lived here together I was surprised that this was the first time I had ever seen one.

After learning a little about the weasel I was wondering if the weasel is what had been after that chicken that was going crazy behind me a little before I seen it for the first time. It would make sense. In what I was reading about weasels, they are really bad for a hen house. So far I haven't seen it around the chicken coop. I really hope it doesn't go there.

Another really cool thing that happens almost every year. I say almost because I only think she missed one year, I'm not sure though. Maybe we missed her. Every year we plant most of the garden around the last week of May give or take. Some of the garden will already be in by then, but not all of it. Every time we plant the second time, about a week later there is a spot in the garden that gets dug up, well actually two spots and a trail to the second spot. We have a snapping turtle that comes back to the exact same spot every year to lay her eggs. After we plant the corn usually she will dig up her first spot with her back feet, or just act like it. We are starting to think that is just a diversion in case a critter was looking to dig up turtle eggs. We say this because she only lays the eggs In the second hole she digs. Both holes are always in the same place, with the exception of the first year we seen her. That year she dug like five holes before she laid her eggs in the exact same spot.

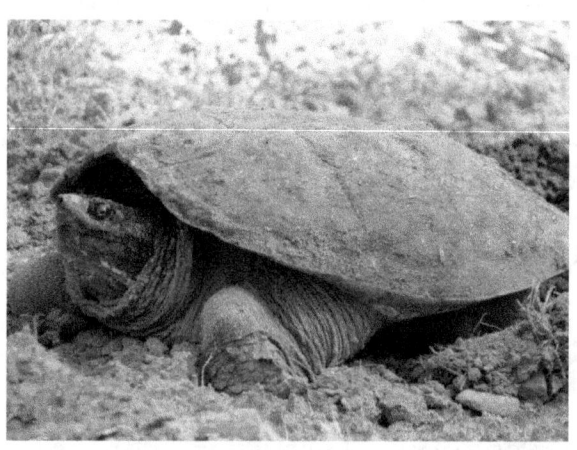

That may have been because when I seen her I was mowing the grass on a riding lawn mower. I'm actually surprised I seen her because the grass had gotten really tall before I mowed it. It was funny because I kept mowing, and she kept hanging around. She would move a little closer to where she needed to be when I wasn't close to her. Then she'd sit and wait to move when I was mowing around her. It took a while to finish the grass because I had to keep going in different circles to avoid her and give her some space. It was kind of comical. I had to finish the grass though, because once the lawn mower got hot and I shut it off it wouldn't start again until the next day. She and I made it through the grass cutting just fine. I didn't figure she would take the lawn mower as well as she did, but it didn't seem to bother her all that much. After I was almost finished she had made it to her preferred spot in our garden and was laying her eggs in the hole she dug.

One year we dug the eggs up and put them in sand in a cage that stayed in the yard close to the garden. We only put them in a cage to prevent another critter from digging up the eggs and eating them. We left the cage in the weather as they would be in nature. We made sure that where we put the cage the eggs would get the same amount of sunlight as where the turtle had buried them and we covered them with about the same amount of sand as the turtle had covered them in dirt. Our cage worked out nicely and we were able to grab all of the fifty babies once they hatched and we took them down to the swamp. I'm not sure how many made it, because we never see any turtles in the swamp, but we're hoping they did.

I always go see her if I am home when she lays her eggs. I take a bunch of pictures and sometimes I try to lay something next to her so we can have an idea her size compared to something that is easy to judge by. This year was no exception, our turtle showed up and I noticed her only after the first mock hole was done and she had already dug the second hole with her back feet and had backed her butt into the hole and was laying her eggs. I had just woke up and was still clearing the sleep from my eyes when I seen the dark spot from our bedroom window across the road in the garden. Then I noticed that dark spot was larger than normal. After wiping my eyes yet again I realized that there was a turkey stomping on that turtles back and he was trying to steal her eggs. With my pistol on my belt, camera around my neck, and my coffee and cigarettes in tow I was off to run that turkey away from our turtle. I jogged all the way across the road yelling and got within eight to ten feet of that turkey before it finally walked away towards the woods. I said hello to my little buddy and snapped a few pictures of her. I always talk to her for a few minutes. She doesn't care if I walk right up to her. She has never been aggressive with me yet. The only thing I have not done is to touch her, I wouldn't want to be rude or invasive. When you have a mutual respect with most animals, you'd be surprised where that leads. She lets me into her space without incident, and I don't push it.

Anyway, I was still half asleep and decided to come back to the house for more coffee before I took some more pictures of the turtle. No sooner than I walked back into the house I heard Joseph yelling to me from upstairs. "Hey! That turkey's back!". I yelled back and told him it wasn't there because I had just run it off. He yelled back to me and said go look again and that it was back. I took off toward the front door and sure enough that turkey was back stomping on the turtles back and trying to get his head in under her butt to eat her eggs. I ran out the front door and was yelling all the way across the road. The turkey did not even flinch until I was almost standing over top of him. He finally waddled off to the woods and I hid behind a tree for quite some time to make sure I could go back for my coffee without the turkey coming right back. I waited there for what seemed like a half hour and no turkey. I headed back for my desperately needed coffee. Once again, guess who had been waiting for me to go away? You guessed it, the turkey. I was almost to the front door when I heard the Nextel beep and I was already doing a u-turn to run that bugger off again. This time I was still without coffee and getting pissed. All I wanted was to grab my coffee cup and I was so close this time! Okay the gloves were off now. I ran across the road, the yard, and the garden again yelling and flailing my arms like a nut case and chased the turkey off again. Only this time I watched closely where it went in and which direction it was heading and away from where the turkey could have been, I fired four rounds from my Sig Sauer 9mm into the woods. This time I went straight for my coffee cup, and I got it. No more turkey. After I got my coffee I spent about another 45 minutes with our turtle before leaving her alone for a while. I mostly stayed back a little ways because I didn't want to disturb her while she was trying to lay her eggs. Her day had been eventful enough. I took a few close up pictures then stepped back and used the zoom lens for the rest. Then I went back up stairs. I kept watching for when she was ready to leave and then ran outside again to take more pictures of her as she was leaving.

Last year we dug up the eggs and put them in an empty aquarium in the house. We did research online to figure out what the best way would be to give them all a chance at hatching. I did everything it said to do and none hatched. When it got to the one hundred and twentieth day mark I was surprised I wasn't seeing any movement. After another month of Joseph telling me the eggs weren't going to hatch and that they had to go, I finally got them out of the house. I felt horrible. I thought I did everything right and that they would hatch. When they didn't I felt as though I had done something terribly wrong with respect to that turtle. She brings her eggs here every year because she apparently feels they are safe here and I let her down. This year when she was finished Joseph and I grabbed one of our famous garden crates and covered that area so nothing could get in to bother her eggs but her babies could get out if they hatched.

Those crates to keep the critters from eating the cabbage and other stuff have now become turtle egg protectors as well. I love this place!

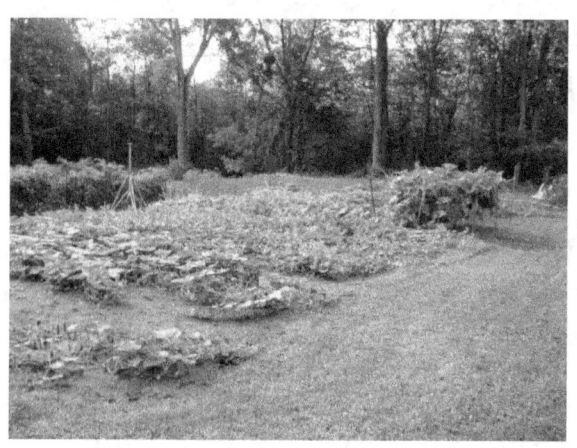

When I was looking up information on how to care for the eggs and the baby turtles I think it said something about the snapping turtle population being very low. I hadn't seen a snapping turtle before living with

Joseph. I hadn't seen one at all in at least twenty years. Reading up on snapping turtles I learned several interesting facts I hadn't known, and would have never thought of. I guess according to this one website, it said something about the temperature average throughout their incubation having something to do with whether the turtles will be males or females. I think it was the temperature as well that could change the amount of days the eggs incubate. I take all I find with a grain of salt, but no matter what it is all food for thought, and yet another reason to watch the nature around here as much as possible to learn all I can from it.

I am looking forward to seeing baby snapping turtles again this fall. They have repeatedly taken one hundred and twenty days to hatch. They always hatch the first or second week of September, depending on which week she lays her eggs in. I think that is awesome because my Grandparents wedding anniversary is on September ninth. Sometimes on their anniversary baby turtles hatch and keep my mind off of the fact that I can't see them near as much as I would like to.

The coolest thing about this turtle is the fact that no matter when she lays her eggs, not matter what is growing, she never hurts anything in our garden. This year our corn was about three to four inches tall when she made her way into the garden. We once again did not lose a single plant to her digging her hole, laying her eggs and tracking in and out of the garden. That's what I mean about living together. She never damages anything in our garden and we watch out for her eggs. There aren't very many snapping turtles around anymore and you don't see many people caring for them. This is yet another way we can give back to nature. Not to mention another testimony to how well humans and wildlife can live together if we choose to. She is another example also of the fact that most wild animals will not bother you if you don't bother them.

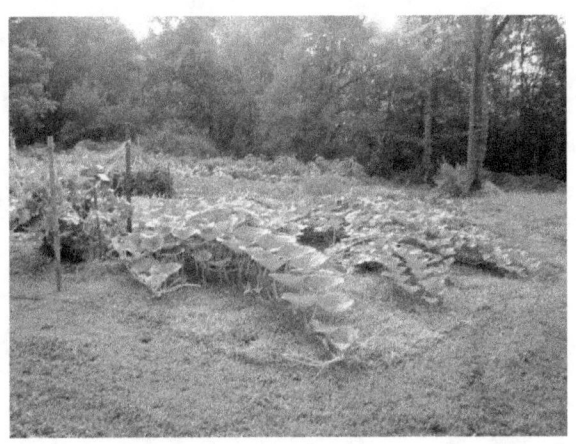

Chapter 9
Canning

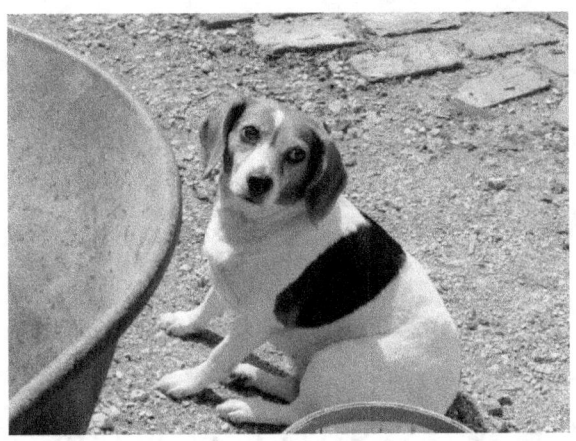

{This is a picture taken while we were bringing in the sweet corn, our beagle was supervising the work.}

I have no intention of trying to explain to anyone how to can here, but I can convey to you what we have learned and maybe a few helpful hints.

When we first started out with our garden, our intention was to be able to both eat out of it all summer long as well as be able to put as much away as possible for the winter months by canning whatever we could.

I have already covered how bad our experiences have been with purchased foods of every kind and the only way to solve that problem was to begin canning as much as possible to hold us over until the next garden season.

We bought a cherry tree, and we have black raspberries berries growing wild everywhere on our property. We met a really sweet lady at a garage sale who offered us some strawberry plants that she had to part with because her strawberry patch was getting too big. She also offered us an established grapevine to transplant. We accepted the offers and we brought the grapevine and a piece of fence it had been growing on as well as the strawberries home. Our intention with the grapevine was to make wine and we both really wanted strawberries. We ate all the strawberries the first year and then I noticed that a mole had tunneled under each and every strawberry plant we had. The following year none of the strawberries had come back up and I was certain the mole had eaten the roots and killed the plants. Is that true, I don't know for sure, but I know it's what I think happened. We ended up buying a slew of strawberry plants again the following year and the exact same thing happened again! Now I was sure that the mole did it. No one else had any problem keeping strawberries, and we knew our soil was good. At least we had planted them in spring and were able to use the berries they produced to can and freeze during time.

In spring the first things to can around here are the wild berries or the strawberries if we have them. Now picking the black raspberries when they are growing everywhere can be quite a challenge. As much as I hate the stuff, there is no getting around using bug spray. I know this from personal experience. I let a friend talk me into trying a dryer sheet to keep the mosquitoes away, only once. It does not work! You can't exactly be swatting bugs away when you are neck deep in thorns and trying to pick berries. Trust me, I know this, it just doesn't work. You end up dropping your berries and bleeding at some point. That is simply unavoidable.

Anyway, we took big bowls with us and began picking berries. It takes quite a few berries to make jelly so it usually takes half the day or more just to pick them. One thing that I have learned is that you should never pick more than you get canned within about a twenty-four hour period. If I couldn't finish canning the jelly today, it would have to be done tomorrow or the berries would be wasted. Fresh fruits and vegetables don't like to be handled and then stacked on top of one another in a bowl, whether they are in the fridge or not. No matter what it is you're canning, the fresher it is the better it will taste when you decide to open the jar.

When you can berries, you have to be aware that the acidity content in them can vary from year to year. When this increases or decreases it changes not only your processing times, but also the amount of sugar you'll need to perfect your recipe. Thanks be to Mamaw for teaching me these little tricks. She saved an entire batch of strawberry jelly for me one year, because I thought it was bad. She explained to me how I could reprocess it and she was right, of course, and I didn't lose any of the strawberry jelly I had made.

Another way to preserve your berries is to freeze them. I did this the first year, but not anymore after that. I don't care for the change in the berries once they are frozen. When you thaw them out they are softer, which is fine for pies, but not for eating fresh. I'm not much on making pies, so I see no need to freeze more than enough to make a pie for Thanksgiving or for Christmas.

If you are thinking about learning to can or freeze produce from your garden, you're going to want to invest about six dollars in what I call my canning bible, it's called the "Ball Blue

Book". Most stores carry this book in the aisle where they sell the other canning supplies like jars and lids, etc. This book is a step by step how-to on what seems to be anything and everything I ever wanted to look up. The only recipe I cannot find and continue to look for is a recipe for pickled eggs. I have wanted to try that for years. My first try was complete failure. We won't go there, even though it was funny.

If I see a garage sale and I spot canning jars, I'll scrape up quarters to buy the darn things. I have a good supply of them right now, but when you do a lot of canning it seems you can never have enough jars. When you are just starting out trying to learn to can and you don't have much money to work with, that can sometimes be the only way you can acquire the jars you need. I remember one year I had no more jars and had plenty of things to can, just not enough money to buy as many jars as I was going to need. I took the money I had to work with and bought enough jars to can what I needed to, then had enough left over for almost the rest of the season just by going to garage sales. Every year we have to by new lids, because those cannot be reused. I use them to cap jars when I use them to hold flour or sugar or something. You just can't reuse them when you are initially preserving your foods.

When a jar has a chip or it can no longer be used for canning for one reason or another, I find alternative uses for them. I have canning jars filled with anything and everything you can imagine. I have them in china cabinets, use them for bugs, even for canisters on the kitchen counter. If one of the jars I get from a garage sale can't be cleaned, then it gets set aside and eventually filled with used or old cooking oils to be thrown away or recycled. We have even used them for drinking glasses. As a matter of fact there is a half gallon jar of iced tea in the fridge right now.

I have an old family recipe for cabbage soup which I absolutely love. Only problem is, when I make it, it takes a big pot and it ties up the fridge for days. Though I love it, you can only eat so much cabbage soup in one weeks time span. When I can my favorite soup I can go to the pantry and open a jar and have it whenever I want without having to make it right then. It always tastes as fresh and just as good as the day I made it. We grow almost all of the ingredients I need for my favorite soup in our garden, so I can have garden fresh cabbage soup any time of the year. Just as easy as using a can opener, but no ingredients I can't pronounce or spell.

I have always loved pickles, and pickles are getting quite expensive these days if you're on a budget. Same thing goes for pickled mild or hot pepper rings, oh how I could eat those by the gallon. All we have to do is grow the cucumbers and the mild peppers and I can usually come up with enough to last for over a year or two in only one season. When you start looking at all of things I don't have on my grocery bill, it adds up to be a lot. That of course depends on how productive the season was that year, and how many critters have shared in our garden goodies and how much they ate.

The nice thing about canning pickles is that they last for a long time once they are canned. Only problem is if it's the first year, you have to wait about six months before you eat them or the pickles won't be all the way pickled yet. I like to keep the pickles on what I call a last year cycle. The pickles

I canned last year will be the ones we'll eat this year. The book will tell you like six weeks or something, but we have found that they are at their optimum flavor after about six months.

Making homemade salsa is another thing we enjoy. If you don't have time to stand in the kitchen and dice up veggies all day, just use a blender. Depends on if you must have chunky salsa, or if you like salsa without big chunks. These are the days when a food processor becomes your best friend. Oh the time it saves. The fingers too if you get in a rush like I do and always manage to hurt yourself in one way or another. Patience and help are two blessed things when you're canning. Having someone else to help with all of the preparation makes the work load much lighter.

It's a good way to spend some good quality time together as well.

Joseph and I, when we can together, spend hours talking and listening to the radio when we are in the kitchen. Having a few beers mixed in there can turn the whole canning event into your own personal party. No matter how you look at it, it is food for the mind, body, and soul. It brings us closer when we spend time canning together.

Usually after the berries are done, the next things to start coming in are either the peppers or the tomatoes. Also the lettuce, cucumbers and green beans. All depends on when and how everything was started. If it was a plant that we transplanted or if it was from seed.

Joseph loves fresh hot peppers, and pickled hot peppers. He has no choice but to help me with those. I can handle and process the cayenne's, just not so much the jalapeños. When I handle them, under my nails will burn for a few days. You are supposed to use rubber gloves when you process hot peppers. I have really small hands and the gloves are always huge and baggy on my fingers. How can you process and cut up peppers like that? I can't, so I just do all I can until I can't handle it anymore and the rest either Joseph does or they wait a while until he has time. It doesn't matter if you scrub your hands in the strongest soap on the market, the oils from those hot peppers will not come off! At least I haven't found a way to get it off yet. It takes several days or more for it to wear off. You learn quick to not touch your eyes or nose, or anything else for that matter, for at least three days when you process hot peppers. Well for people like me anyway. Joseph is fine by the next day. I guess everyone is different in that respect. I guess my aunt ended up in the hospital once with burns on her hands from the hot peppers. Like I said everyone is different. So if you process hot peppers just be careful and take proper precautions until you know your boundaries or you may be sorry later.

The cucumbers and peppers usually go fairly quickly because you don't have to use the pressure canner for those. You can use a water bath canner which only takes 15 minutes to process the jars. The pressure canner takes longer because it has to build and maintain pressure for the amount of minutes that recipe takes to complete. You must follow pressures and times to the letter, if you don't it can cause bacteria in the jars or even botulism. Everything has to be clean and sterile and done properly. This is serious business and cleanliness is extremely important. That is one area to never compromise or cut corners on.

You also can't use metal utensils in jars or during the filling of the jars. You need wooden or plastic utensils. All of those important pointers are included in that Ball Blue Book I was telling you about earlier. If you are trying to learn to can, definitely read that book before you begin actually canning anything and understand what your utensils need to be and all of the do's and don'ts. Canners require special care and there are some cleaners that should never be used on a canner.

When you get toward the latter days of your garden you can use small portions of this and that to create different types of sauces, dressings, or relishes. This comes in handy when you don't have enough of one thing to can a jar of just that, but you don't want to waste it either. The possibilities are truly endless, and nothing but your imagination can limit you.

When canning season gets close I usually have to go stock up on vinegar.

That is one thing we go through what seems like a metric ton of throughout the canning season. Just recently I went to the store and brought home twelve big jugs of vinegar and a pack of Zippo flints. That took every penny I had in my pocket, and the look on the cashiers face was hilarious!

Canning is both fun and healthy, as long as you do it correctly that is. Another great advantage to canning your own recipes is that what you can is made the way you like it. Not the way it was mass produced. There is only one thing I have purchased from the store that I don't open and totally change what it started as by adding this, that or the other thing. I can't remember who makes it, but it's spaghetti sauce and it comes in tomato & basil and other combinations I can't remember at the moment. If you peel the label off it is packed in a mason jar! That is some of the best sauce I have ever had. When I have to buy sauce because we are out of what I have canned, that is the only kind I want. It has flavor, which in my opinion is hard to find in anything from a store these days. I have to go look right now and find out what kind of sauce that was, because it has just got to be mentioned here. Hold on...okay got it, it's called "Classico". If you can't can, or don't want to can, but really want some real flavor that tastes like home grown, then you have to try that sauce. No, nobody paid me to say that, I'm just so amazed that there is one thing from the store that actually tastes like it was picked this morning and made fresh this afternoon.

You can also can meats and virtually anything else you can think of. I hope you can and do can. Ha! That sounded funny. Seriously though I do. You'll be doing yourself and your family a great service to their health and well being if you do. Your grocery bill will shrink drastically as well. You can't lose.

That reminds me, I have a counter full of tomatoes screaming my name right now, and green beans are waiting for me in the garden. Wahoo!

Chapter 10
Canning Stories

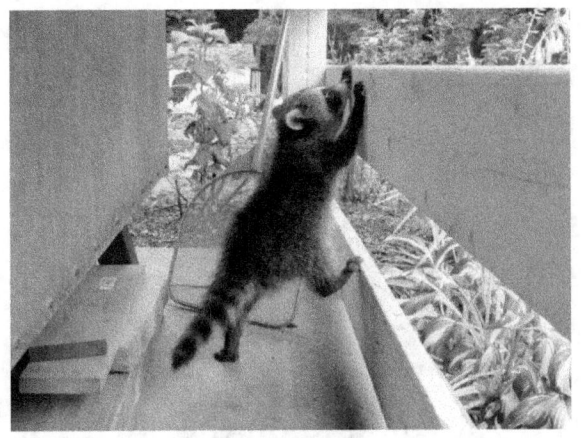

{This is a picture of a raccoon on the porch.}

This is canning so there isn't much to be told in the way of stories. Well, except for one. A few years back I was just overwhelmed with canning to get done and I didn't have any real help that year. I was getting frustrated and in too much of a hurry trying to keep up with work, the weeding, the picking, and the preparing and canning of food for the winter. We might remind you of squirrels packing their nest with food for the winter.

I was making spaghetti sauce and had a large pot cooking on the stove. It was done and I had begun to fill my hot jars to preserve the sauce. I had this bad habit of holding the jars up by the top and using the ladle to fill the jars. I very often spilled the sauce, or whatever else it was I was canning at the time on my hand. This day was no different, and at this point I had already burned my hand about five or six times. I just learned to grin and bear it, grit my teeth and finish what I was doing until I could set it down. I was not going to let a jar drop and waste all of that good food or hard work for that matter. I wasn't far into starting to can this big pot of sauce when I burned my hand again. Only this time I had spilled just enough sauce on my hand for it to get between my fingers and the jar and cause me to lose my grip.

At the time I was wearing a pair of my favorite jeans that are now shorts. There were holes in both the knees and the upper thighs of both legs of these jeans, and the holes were not by any means small. We rarely had extra money to go clothes shopping, and I am known to use something until it is physically impossible to use it any further. These jeans were no exception to my rule. I had only had them for about year or a little more at that point, and wasn't happy I had spent all that money to finally buy new jeans and they were in such bad shape so quickly. Like I said they were my favorite most comfy jeans and I was not giving them up until I had no other choice. I wasn't kidding when I said they are now shorts. By this time Joseph had been bugging me for quite a while to get rid of my ratty jeans. I had already told him a thousand times that I would not part with them until I absolutely had to and to quit complaining about the holes in them because it would do no good. I loved those jeans, they were staying, and that was that. As you get older it does become more about cost and comfort, at least for me anyway.

When that sauce came between my hand and that jar, the jar was full of boiling spaghetti sauce. Now in a perfect world the jar would have fallen away from me and my holy jeans and landed on the stove and made a huge mess. In my world it dumped right down the front of me. Starting just below my waist and filling every giant hole in both legs of my favorite jeans. I had a quart mason jar full of sauce in my hand when it dumped down the front of me, and very little of that sauce landed on the floor. When it hit my legs I was not sure if I was going to scream, pass out, or cry. There were younger kids in the house so I couldn't just rip my pants off like I wanted too and all I could say was; "oh shit!". I turned in circles couple times and ran upstairs to rip the jeans off. Now I only ran upstairs at this point because I had hot jars waiting and jars processing in the water bath canner. Joseph came to check on me because he is always so worried something will happen to me. He is somewhat overprotective I guess. I told him to man the sauce for me until I could change my pants. All of that boiling sauce that had been caught in those giant holes of my favorite pants that I had refused to give up and it was extremely painful. I quickly changed into a pair of shorts, peeling the sauce and my skin off with my jeans, and headed back downstairs to tend to my sauce. Joseph was amazed when he saw my legs. He said we needed to go to the hospital right that minute. I argued and said it would calm down in a little while like anything else and I wasn't wasting all of these vegetables from the garden. I had to finish canning them and I wasn't going anywhere until that was done. After a few minutes the pain from any injury tends to lessen and then you can get on with whatever it was that you were doing. I am here to tell you that burns are whole different beast. The pain did not subside, not even a little. Joseph helped me finish canning and then took me to the emergency room. It had been a couple hours and the pain hadn't let up one bit. I had hoped a few beers would help, but no such luck. So off the emergency room we went.

I waited in the emergency room for I think three or four hours. I tried blowing on the burns and even that hurt. Now I know I'm goofy, and I also know this woman meant well, but... A lady walked up to me after I had been there a couple hours. It is hard to not take deep breaths and try to fan a burn. The pain was almost overwhelming and had still not let up at all. This lady asked me if I wanted an ice pack for my leg. She didn't look like a nurse, thank god, and god bless her for wanting to try to help someone, but the last thing someone with a burn wants is to put an ice pack or anything else on exposed nerves and dangling scorched flesh!

I finally got to see the doctor and she gave me some pain medication and this cream that about took my breath away when she applied it to the burns. I had second and third degree burns over about twenty to thirty percent of my right leg. My left leg had only red spots and no actual burns and by this time the redness was beginning to fade some on my left leg. That cream seemed to help numb and cool the area when the pain killers kicked in. I only had a third degree burn on a small part of my right leg, and I only know this because that was the only area that had no feeling when I poked it. Wearing jeans at this point was completely out of the question, and I had to work in the morning. I went to work in the same pair of bright purple baggy pants for over a week because I couldn't wear anything else. Those purple pants ended up being the only thing we owned between the both of us that I could wear over those burns. I don't own sweat pants and I wasn't allowed to wear shorts to work, not that I would have that week anyways. After about a week I was better able to move around and wear my normal clothes over the bandages on my leg. After a month it had finally healed enough to forget about it for the most part.

After about a year it had healed so well that you couldn't see even a trace of any of the scars I had. It had healed beautifully. I had not expected that and was quite happy because the scars would have been rather large.

Though canning for the most part can be rather uneventful, never let your guard down and always be careful!

Chapter 11
Hunting

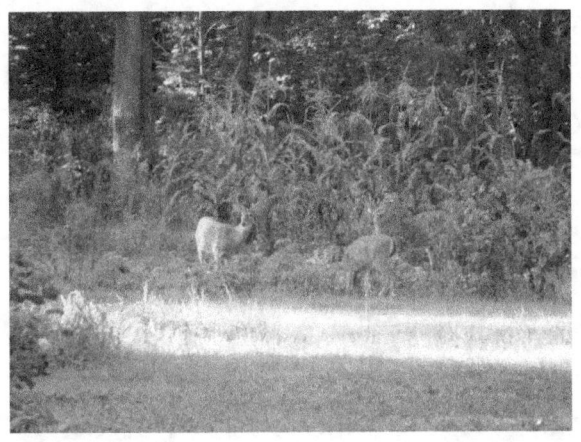

{This is a picture of our garden and the four deer who were dining there one morning. Only two of the four deer can be seen in this picture.}

I'm going to start here by saying I was raised by a hunter and so was Joseph. When we hunt, we are ethical hunters who are not haphazardly running around like idiots with guns and bows in the woods. We don't spend our time out in the woods to be able to come back and brag to our friends and we don't come back shouting bullshit stories just so we can sound cool to morons who find that sort of thing interesting. We are real and in tune with our natural habitat around us. We are also both of strong Native American decent and believe in honoring the beings who give themselves to us for our nourishment and sustenance.

Mostly what we hunt is white tail deer. I love rabbit and squirrel, but with how busy we stay there just isn't enough time to spend cleaning and skinning the smaller animals for what little amount of meat we can get from them. Every now and then I make extra time to do so, but not very often.

Every year we purchase as many permits as we are permitted by law. We need on average about six to seven average size deer to feed us for the rest of the year if we do not have hogs that year. If we end up with a larger deer, then we don't need as many deer that year. We don't hunt until we fill all of our tags. We hunt until we have met our quota for what will feed our family until the next season and no more. Take from the Earth what is needed and nothing more; these are words to live by.

We process our own deer. The reason we do this is because when you drop your deer off at the butcher, you may or may not get your deer back. I like the way our deer around here taste because of the diets they consume in our area. I know that we have properly field dressed our deer and we have not tainted any meat. I don't want someone else's anything because I don't know where it has been, how it has been kept, or how it has been handled. There are a great many people out there who don't wash the meat because they say it changes it. Well son you can keep your dirty unwashed meat all to yourself. I want no part of that. Not a single person has ever complained about any of the meat they have eaten here, even if they did I probably wouldn't care. If it hasn't been rinsed off and cleaned I won't cook it.

To be quite honest I don't like the way a commercially processed deer is done. The fat and sinew are not removed from the meat as we do. The gristle in a deer is not what we want in our meals.

When we field dress a deer we immediately hang it up and rinse it out with the hose. If it is early in bow season, when the weather is warmer, the deer won't hang long and gets rinsed out often until we begin to process it.

The first thing we do is skin the deer. Once the skin is free I set it aside to be cleaned further and salted. When we are ready to process our deer many things happen. I thoroughly clean all of the counters and the sink in the kitchen. As I said we are poor folk so we have to make due any way we can. I bring out clean bowls and knives, then we begin. As we begin to remove parts, they are placed in bowls. Each time the bowl is full I take it to the kitchen and rinse it well. Being certain to remove any dirt, debris, and any hair. It is then set on a pitched porcelain sink to drain. I head back out for more. Once the sink is full and I still have more meat to be rinsed, we set the pieces in a clean cooler to be sure no flies can get to the meat and that it will be cool until we get to it. Then I finish any rinsing and cleaning.

With the meat set off to the side of the sink we have room to clean everything we just used as well as wash our hands. We have a meat grinder that you churn by hand and that is washed and set in place before we begin the last stages of processing. All the clean damp and dry rags are set out. The pans and bowls to collect the different cuts of meat are clean and ready. The packing area is ready and so are we. The radio will be on and a beer with a straw is set out so that our hands will remain sterile while we are processing.

Joseph does the steak cuts and the processing of all of the meat that gets cut from the bone. When he has a full bowl I come and take it and rinse it again and then I package it. Unless of course it is meat that needs to be ground into burger. Then it only gets rinsed a second time if there is some reason that requires it. If that is not the case then I begin to grind the meat. When the meat is ground I take it to the packing area and grab what is needed to fill the freezer paper with ground meat and then I fold it, tape it up, and label it.

I am the one who keeps the counters and rags clean as he does all of the important processing. When I am done packaging or pre-cleaning the meat he is cutting up, I take to wiping things off and making sure he has what he needs to keep the area clean and as sterile as humanly possible. I change the rags and sometimes wash or rinse the knife. I set out fresh paper towels and anything else that needs to be addressed.

Next of the things that deserve mention here is the squirrels and the rabbits. Now I absolutely love rabbit and squirrel meat. Just as much as I love pheasant and turkey and quail and just about any other wild game you pass my way. I have no problem cleaning it and eating it. If I had more time I would eat a lot more squirrel than I do. I just simply do not have enough time to work the garden and wrestle with small game and contend with everything else that gets put on my plate at home. I really wish I did, but I don't.

I've also been told recently that ground hog is good eatin'. Once again, if I had the time to kill, skin, and process it, I darn sure would eat it. It is a vegetarian so it must taste pretty darn good. One thing I would never eat is an Opossum. They eat left over dead stuff, road kill, or they will kill and eat chickens. All I know is that vegetarians taste better from the wild. I would also eat a raccoon if I had to, I have also heard those aren't bad either, I'd give it a try.

Now don't start on that "oh they are so cute I wouldn't eat them" trip because if you were hungry enough you'd probably eat the asshole out of a cat. And in other countries the things we snub our noses at are delicacies, so get real. No, you may not like how it sounds. Someday you just may be depending on what you are freaking out over today. Anyone want a chocolate covered grasshopper?

Once again I will reiterate the fact that animals were put here for us to thrive from. Should you decide to be a vegetarian, well more power to you I suppose. But do not expect hunters like me to support your view. The only difference between hunters and vegetarians in my opinion is the fact that a hunter won't force their opinions down your damn throat and tell you that you need to start hunting and eating meat. We aren't like vegetarians who think we have to convert the world. I have yet to meet a vegetarian that did not begin by telling me how meat does this and that to a person's body. I hunt, I eat meat, and I don't rightly care what an anti meat eater wants to tell me, I'm going to keep killing it and eating it. A real hunter won't ever show their face on TV and tell everyone they must eat meat or they are anti-earth. Real hunters aren't PETA assholes who think it's acceptable to destroy another's belongings or attack another human being to justify their cause. Real hunters are real people, with real values and families who would never treat other human beings in such a crude and belligerent fashion.

Take my opinion for what it is or leave it, I don't care. But I will not have some bunch of gossiping bitches telling me I cannot live as my ancestors did. For the time being we are blessed with living on seventy acres and will treat it no differently than our ancestors did prior to us. We will hunt it efficiently and correctly. We will not over hunt this land no matter what the circumstance and we will protect this domicile with our lives. More people should understand what it is to *properly* manage the wildlife on this amount of acreage and any other amount of acreage. That simple.

Another thing, don't act like I'm stupid and tell me to eradicate the doe population because you are too stupid to see that the human race has over populated their area. Not the other way around! I am not a horn hunter and do not see the need in this new bullshit theory to talk to hunters and hope they will let the small bucks go and start eliminating the doe in hopes to cut the population and create bigger better bucks. What you will create with that is an unstable population of deer with an uncertain future should any small problem arise in the deer population.

All of your shitty hunters will never do it right if they weren't already doin' it right! The only people that are affected by feeding restrictions and culling are the average people hoping to eat some real meat from the wild and most likely to help with the grocery bill. I know from personal experience and from actually paying attention to the wildlife around us what works to properly manage our property to ensure the deer population. Don't be selfish or take their habitat. The human population needs to look at their own invasive over population of wildlife habitat. Hunting started out as a way for people to sustain themselves. Before grocery stores became the only place many people have ever seen meat.

I have hated over the years watching the people in the hunting community that only hunt for horns, poach, and trespass give the sport and the people who respect the sport a bad name.

It makes me mad when I hear of insurance companies and other people crying because they say the deer population is too high.   I say different. I used to see herds of deer coming through our property at about fifteen to twenty each passing at a minimum. Now I'm lucky to see two or three. What that tells me is the insurance companies are full of shit and big business just wants us more dependent on them than on any natural resource we may have once had before poor management practices. Before too many wooded areas were cleared for housing. Back when there was still enough room for the wildlife to live without being noticed because their habitat was still intact enough for them to survive without being noticed by humans.

Okay, this is obviously a subject close to my heart and one I don't take kindly to anyone screwing with! Especially when it involves decisions made by authorities that are seemingly made with a complete lack of common sense. In those instances I often wonder which billion dollar industry bought that law.

No matter how you view it, we can live off of a trivial amount of land and sustain ourselves if we just choose to get off of our rear ends and do so. As long as we pay attention to the impacts of our decisions on the surrounding wildlife populations and understand the natural world around us. As long as people cooperate with hunters trying to find the animal they have harvested and now need to locate. As long as everyone does things in an ethical and respectful manner there should be no problems. Am I in a dream world? Maybe I am, but one can always have hope.

That's all I have to say about that.

Chapter 12
Hunting Stories

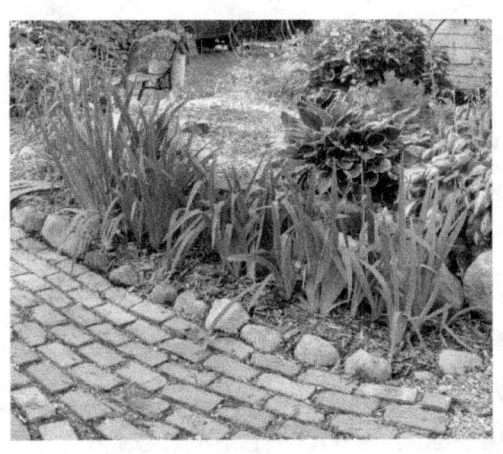

{This is a picture of a portion of a flower bed and the brick walk way we built to walk around it.}

Joseph and I are both hunters. The difference is, he has been hunting for years and I haven't. I didn't have a place to hunt before we got together and I had (still have) no intentions of hunting on state land. The first year we were together I wanted to start white tail deer hunting. As it turned out a guy I had been working with was in need of money and was selling an old PSE Polaris Express bow for fifty dollars. I bought it. Joseph showed me how to tune the bow in and make sure everything was safe and in sync as it should be.

In case you haven't already noticed I'm not too concerned with proper names and labels for pretty much anything except tools. Other than that everything is a thingamabob to me. Regardless of that fact, Joseph showed me how to set my bow up to prepare to shoot. I had a couple months before bow season opened and we began target practicing and sighting in my bow. My first shot was in the target area, and it didn't take long from there to sight it in. I spent a couple weeks fine tuning it and shooting as much as my arm would let me. It took a little while for me to learn how to stop letting the string smack my forearm when I released an arrow. I got much advice, sometimes too much for my liking. When Joseph and I target practice we usually practice together. We watch each other shoot and when we see something that doesn't look right we point it out to each other. I think that is very helpful when you shoot a bow. When I started, I was shooting forty pounds or so I think, and by the end of the season I had graduated to shooting fifty-five pounds, which was where that bow topped out at. I knew I was ready for my first deer when I started hitting my arrows that I had already shot into the target because that bow was so nice to shoot and so deadly accurate. The arrows hit their mark with a good thump.

We went out hunting together every time we hunted. He was going to show me the ins and outs of hunting. I was happy we were out hunting together and I was itching to get a chance to take my first shot at a deer. We had this tree stand that would hold the both of us comfortably, and that is where we always went. Later it would become my tree stand and he would practically insist that I hunt from there because the hunting was better from that stand. It was well hidden and had great shooting lanes. The view from that stand was perfect. On our way to the stand one day we seen dumb and dumber. These two little bucks were so funny. They didn't run off when they seen us, they wanted to hang around. While Joseph was playing around with them I was attempting to get a shot off at one of them. They were too far out for me to have a chance and he was so close to them I didn't know how he expected to draw his bow. Then again you never know. He was no more than ten yards away from these two bucks. They were four point bucks and they looked like they were identical twins. They were stomping their feet and snorting at Joseph and I was standing back watching and laughing the whole time. They were fun to mess with, we only seen them a few more times after that day, then we stopped seeing them. I'm sure someone shot them or they got hit by a car. One of the two for sure I would guess.

When we met dumb and dumber we were about a week into bow season I think. By now we had gone out several times and had no luck yet. As well as more than one event like the dumb and dumber incident. Joseph likes to try new things and interact with nature as much as I do. By this time I was getting impatient though and really wanted to be able to take my first serious shot at a deer. I found myself telling him to quit squirming and moving when we were in our tree stand because of my impatience. He was kind of amused with this, but he went along with it anyway being the good sport he is. On this particular day when we were heading out to go hunting, I had told him to save his playing around with the critters until after I got a chance to take my first shot at a live deer and not a target. He agreed. This season was rather warm in October and that is why he hadn't been really serious about taking anything up until now. Nothing had been coming through and it had been unusually hot for that time of year. To leave a deer hang in that kind of heat would not have been good. We had to be prepared to both take it and process it right away. We both had four tags to fill and would be set for the year once the season got going. When we got up in our stand that day he was quite compliant for my sake. I was extremely anxious to take my first shot. Luckily by now we were a couple weeks into the season and the weather had cooled down some which really helped. Joseph had decided that he would not hunt that day and that he would only help me. All he did was rattle and call for me and look out for anything that may possibly have been coming in.

Then he poked me and whispered that a buck was coming our way. Joseph had rattled and here he was, coming across the field and headed right for our tree. It was a six point buck and he was just about to come into the tree line where I wanted him to. Just before that buck went behind that last little tree before entering the tree line where I was, I had drawn my bow and was ready for when he came through on my side. I waited for him to take two steps away from the tree, he gave me the perfect broad side shot and I let my arrow fly. When it hit I knew right then and there that I had a perfect shot. That thwack sound I heard, even though I had never heard it before, was unmistakable. I had seen my arrow hit exactly where it needed to. I started jumping up and down and told Joseph "I hit him, I hit him"! Joseph grabbed me and said that I had better quit before I jump out of the damn tree! I was so excited and was ready to get down but he said no. He informed me that the proper thing to do is wait at least thirty minutes to an hour before getting down to make sure you don't run the deer any farther away than it has already gone. This will greatly increase your likelihood of recovering your deer and help in not wasting that deer's life for no reason. Right then thirty minutes seemed to me as an eternity.

We got down shortly after that and headed in the opposite direction as quietly as possible towards the house. Once we got to the house we gathered flashlights and knives and rags and realized we needed batteries. To keep me occupied long enough, Joseph took me to the twenty-four hour grocery store down the road where we got batteries for the flashlights to be sure we would have more than enough light for the night. I must have looked like redneck on crank at that grocery store. Whatever that would look like I'm not sure. I have a feeling I would have been just that. I was so ready to explode with excitement and still in full hunting garb while walking through the store looking for batteries. I got several strange looks, but I guess no one called the police so I couldn't have been that bad.

If ever there were an easy deer to track, this one was it. Once Joseph picked up where the blood trail began it was an easy walk to where he had come to rest. When I say easy, I mean tracking easy, not actually easy to walk. I had taken my first shot at a deer and had landed my arrow exactly on the mark where it needed to be, the heart, to be able to make a clean and ethical kill. Where he had come to rest was down in a ravine. Not only was the hill steep, it was also covered with trees. He ended up being a six point buck with a body so huge it took everything we had to pull him up the hill and load him into my little S-10 pick-up. This deer was so huge that we were able to keep ribs, and good ribs to say the least. We yielded more meat from this one deer than we normally do when we harvest two and sometimes even three deer. I was, and still am, very proud to have been fortunate enough to be the one that was able to harvest that deer.

After that I was on my own. Joseph knew I was not only able, but quite capable of hunting and he had no more worries of leaving me to my own devices in the field. From there I went on to fill almost all of the rest of my tags that year. I harvested one doe and one more buck. After all of the years I have been hunting, all of the deer except my first one tend run together and I lose track of when and where they were taken. It sounds bad, but between the two of us we have about three sometimes four tags each per year, and that adds up pretty quick. We don't always fill all of the tags if we don't need to. How much we hunt depends on how much meat we have already have and how much more we need. Also on how much meat we yield for each deer we have taken. Also on whether or not we have chosen to take a somewhat smaller deer because it needed to be removed from the herd. Sometimes it is necessary to sacrifice a tag for the good of the herd as well.

One year Joseph took this nice seven point buck with a decent size body, and after we field dressed him and hung him up we realized that he had a severe infection on his back next to his spine. Looking further we found where someone had taken a shot and had horribly missed their mark. I'm not saying that it will never happen to me, but it is only right to do everything in your power to prevent a shitty shot from leaving your arrow rest or your trigger finger. Wasting meat is far worse than passing up the shot entirely, doesn't matter how big or small the deer is. Better to let it walk than to wound it and waste the animal and the meat.

During one of the times that Joseph and I were hunting together out of that tree stand we both used to hunt from, we had quite a unique encounter. We were standing up there scouring the tree lines for movement when we both caught a glimpse of a shadow over our heads. We were both slowly looking anywhere we could through the leaves of that huge Oak tree to try to see what it was that had shadowed us. We couldn't see very much at all and then it was almost right in our faces. It was a Great Horned owl. This Owl had swooped in and landed on the branch that our tree stand was resting on and was only about two feet out from our feet on that branch, if even that far from us. We slowly looked at each other and then back to the Owl. We couldn't believe our eyes. This Owl was so huge and majestic and it was just sitting there looking around. I think that Owl sat with us for probably ten minutes or more. Then it bobbed it's head a couple times, it flew down, grabbed a field mouse, then continued across to the other side of the field and out of sight.

Hunting can be viewed by many people as many things. In my book, if you haven't connected with nature somehow or someway during your adventures into the woods, then I would have to ask if you are missing something. I have just as much fun watching and enjoying the natural world in its natural state when I am hunting as I do when I am blessed enough to be able to harvest a deer.

One minor technicality of living in the woods is learning to exist with the wildlife that surrounds you. It is not always easy, but we do the best we can to survive ourselves without imposing on the habitat that surrounds us.

When I first moved in with Joseph he had (and still have) flower beds. He enjoys flowers as much as I do, so we began to refurbish the old flower beds from years past as well as to build new ones. We have a huge selection of flowers in our yard and our flower beds are huge.

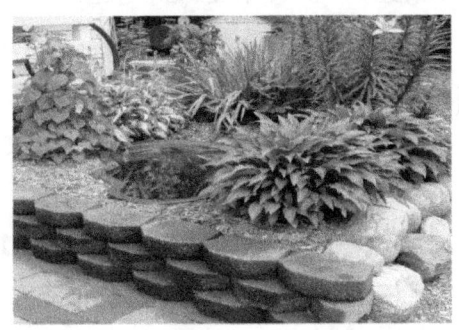

{This is another flower bed with more brick and stone work around it.}

At first we used to have problems with deer walking up and eating the tops off of the flowers. The deer were so bold they would literally walk up to the house and eat the flowers from around the porch area after they had already eaten what they wanted from all of the other flowers beds. On one hand it was kind of funny that they would almost walk across the front porch, but on the other we wanted to see our flowers bloom. We started looking into sprays that claim to keep the deer away and out of your flowers or your garden. At the time I had been working for someone who was having the same problem. It was ironic because he was explaining to me the amount of money he had spent on sprays and other so called deer repellants and he had no luck up to that point deterring the deer from eating his flowers. We didn't have a lot of money to work with and that is all I had to hear to look for another solution. I had started using the dog hair and human hair around the flower beds first to see if it would work. It did work. The deer stopped eating our flowers and for the first time in a couple years we actually got see our tulips and lilies bloom.

When you are lucky enough to be able to hunt at home it's a good thing that the deer are always around. Only problem being all of the things they like to get into when it's not hunting season. Learning to live with them in the off season is always one adventure after another. We all somehow have managed to get along together and it works well for us. Sometimes the best remedy is a cheap and easy one that is right under your nose. I love natural things that work. That is just one less chemical being thrown into our environment and into our watersheds.

No matter what anyone says, we as humans have invaded the living rooms of the natural world to make our homes. The least we can do is offer respect to the animals we must now live with because we have stolen their land out from under them. That is what makes me a better hunter. I know each time I venture into the woods that I am essentially in their living rooms. They know their homes as well as I know mine. They know when someone has entered who doesn't belong. The sooner humans understand that, the sooner they understand how to become better hunters and better care takers of our Earth.

Chapter 13
Raising Pigs

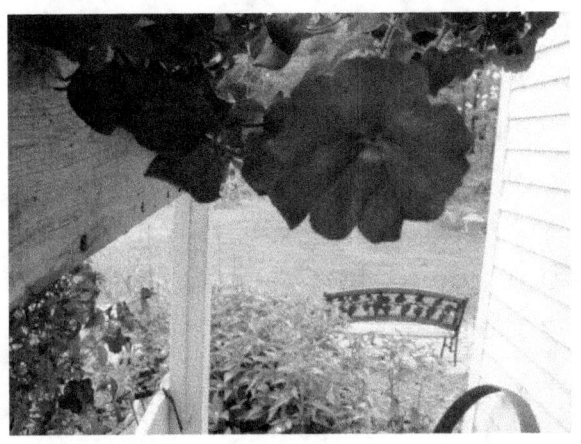

{This is a view of the bench we have on one of the brick walkways and a cute little flower poking out of a hanging planter on the front porch.}

Raising pigs is an absolute necessity in our book. Joseph and I both did purchase bacon and sausage from the store. I have always loved bacon and Joseph has always loved sausage. Joseph raised hogs when he was young. I had never experienced the taste of a home grown hog. Joseph began to talk about raising hogs more and more after the first few years we were together, and he kept telling me how good it was. I knew he had to be right because it only made sense. As soon as we could squeeze the money out of our budget we started calling around for farmers from whom we could purchase a pig. Then a couple years after we started our garden we began raising hogs.

Our first batch of hogs we sent in for butcher told us why we wanted so badly to raise our own. So many people had told us that we were doing it all wrong because our hog pen was too large. We just laughed at them inside and said whatever. If you want to raise a big chunk of fat you can't eat then you go right on ahead.

A hog is not meant to be pinned up in a four foot by five foot area and then slaughtered when it has been fed enough hormones or steroid and antibiotic laced feed to say that it is of slaughter weight. Oh no, no, no, no! What do you eat from an animal? Yes, the meat you eat is the muscle that animal has accumulated. So, what good does it do to pen that animal up and just fatten it up in a cubicle until it is of slaughter weight? NONE! You don't eat the fat, you eat the healthy muscle that animal has gained from running around and being raised correctly. It takes longer and costs more money to raise any animal the right way. To me that is one big DUH! This is where I get pissy (go figure, me pissy?).

An Animal was meant to be harvested for the meat that it provides to the person it gives itself to. We buy our hogs, but our hogs have one hell of a happy life while they are here with us, and yes, then they go to slaughter. We honor our hogs by treating them right while we have them. That simple.

Hogs don't need a huge area, but they do need to be able to run around. Exercise makes muscle and muscle makes meat. Our hogs always end up acting just like the dogs. We just had another hog escape the pen the other day, and she walked right back in when I stood off to the side of the door. They all come up to the gate and tell you when they are hungry. They will also wait for you to scratch their noses, and sometimes their backs.

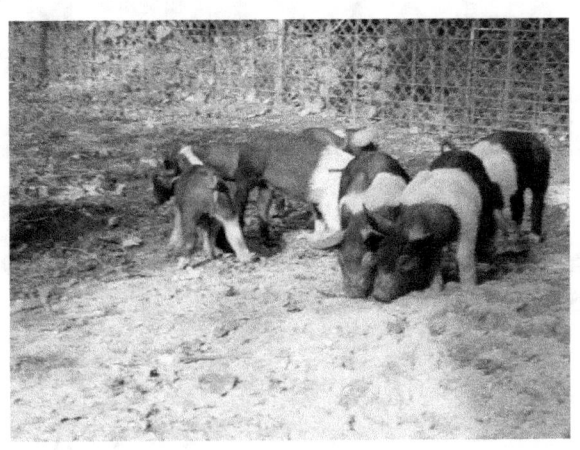

As I'm sure you have noticed, I'm not real concerned with all of the proper names for the pigs at the different stages in their lives. Pig, hog, piglet, sow, and the many others, I don't rightly care. Knowing proper names doesn't make us better able to raise our pigs. I may sound less like a hillbilly, but that doesn't concern me either.

We bought a book on raising pigs when we started, we were looking for insight on symptoms or anything noticeable that would be reason for alarm. When we would need a vet and things like that. So far our pigs have been fairly easy to raise. They mostly just require food (and lots of it), water (and lots of that too), and play time.

We do worm our hogs but we make sure it is quite a while before they go in for slaughter. I don't like chemicals and medicines, especially shortly before they are to be butchered. Unfortunately we must worm them at least once, so we allow time after the worming for the chemicals to leave their systems before they get shipped in. I will only worm them once at the half way point of raising them and that's it. Never had a problem with that so I have no intention of changing the way we handle it.

You haven't really had bacon until you have had bacon from a real home grown hog. It takes me about three pounds of bacon to get enough grease just to make one batch of breakfast gravy! Our hogs are so lean and healthy the meat doesn't produce hardly any grease at all. No-one can tell me that our pork is bad for us.

I always ask for the lard from our hogs. I guess it is not something they just give you back, they ask you if you want it. I'll take it and render it in the oven and use the grease for cooking. The left over chunks after rendering the lard become dogs treats. I would love to make pig skins fresh. I have a feeling they would be really good. When Joseph was growing up his family used to make real pig skins from the hogs they slaughtered. Maybe we'll try that this year. One year I tried to make my own salt pork for pinto beans. It didn't turn out too bad, but I still have some work to do on that recipe before I get that one completely right.

When we raise the hogs we will usually raise anywhere from four to six at a time. Anymore it is getting harder and harder to find someone to buy the pigs from. Many of the pig farms we have seen are now corporation farms and all of their hogs are under contract. I guess when that's the case, the farmers can't sell them or do anything except what the corporation they work for says they can. We were so desperate to find hogs one year that we stopped at several farms and asked if we could buy any pigs, and that is what we were told. That all of the livestock is under contract and that none would be sold. I hadn't realized until then just how many farms had disappeared or been pigeon holed into becoming corporation farms. That is wrong for anyone to allow to happen to any good farmer! Our legislative wonders up on capitol hill want to delegate everything in our lives for us. Now they want to control the food. They should be doing much more to preserve the farmers and their way of living. Not encouraging the sale of their land because big business has driven the prices too low for them to even think of surviving without selling off the very land they have used to sustain themselves and their communities on. I only have one word to describe the feelings I feel when I think of that injustice. Sad!

In an ideal world a person who has a place, be it small or large, to raise livestock could also allow others to keep hogs at their place so more people can share in raising their own food. Most times for the person with the room to do so, that is not worth the hassle. Many people begin raising what they have only for themselves. I think having pigs around is fun, but it still involves work just the same.

It is quite demanding in some respects to have livestock. You have to make sure the coyotes don't get to your animals and kill them. You also have to clean the pen and feed and water them daily. As they get bigger you have you feed them twice a day. That is where having an automatic feeder would be very nice. When you are poor, you work harder for what you have because you can't afford the luxuries that make life easier. I am fine with that because what doesn't kill you will most certainly make you stronger. Someday I hope to have, not only an automatic feeder, but an automatic water spout as well. You also need to inspect the fencing often. Hogs like to root around and some days we wonder if they aren't trying to dig to China. Hogs are also very good at tearing things up. They are very strong animals. We have spent a good deal of time shoveling dirt back into holes to make sure they don't escape and mending the fence. They also tear up the shelter we made for them, and that is no easy repair. Anything new in a hog pen is nothing more than a hog target. I have to look at it this way, if I wasn't outside working, then what else would I be doing? This way I stay busy and out of trouble. Unlike the hogs we raise who are always looking for any trouble they can root their little noses into.

Going on summer vacations is out of the question around here though. If my family lived closer to me, I would never complain about the lack of time for vacations. I am quite content to stay home and enjoy all of the animals and the garden. You have to enjoy the simple things in life to live they way we do.

When all is said and done and the hogs have reached their ideal weight then we have to make phone calls to set appointments with the appropriate people. I think it works out in the end to be somewhere a little above two dollars per pound to raise and have the hogs butchered. Much of the hog meat is smoked, and the sausage gets mixed to the flavor we choose. We get the spicy bulk sausage because that is the only way we can have the sausage and be sure we are getting our own meat back. The butcher that does our hogs does such a great job. The smoked hams are excellent. We send our hogs in when they reach about two hundred-thirty pounds or so. On an average we will get anywhere from one hundred-sixty to one hundred-ninety pounds of meat back per hog. The bill per hog is usually anywhere from one hundred and fifty dollars to two hundred and seventy dollars depending on the cuts of meat we selected for that hog and how much is to be smoked. When we take four hogs in at the end of the year the bill can be a little high to pay all at once. Break that down and do some math and you'll still come out a lot or at least a little ahead of the grocery stores. In all reality you can't really compare the quality of our meat to that of any store. You can't buy meat as pure and healthy and we raise it anywhere that I have ever heard of. Also, don't forget to factor in how much money you have spent in feed, and then you can find the average cost per pound to raise your own pork. Even if it were more to raise our own I still believe it would be well worth it. No, I know for certain it would be well worth it!

Before the corn prices went way up I had the average cost per hog to raise from start to finish figured at between three hundred dollars and four hundred dollars each if I figured it correctly. Not including the butchering cost, but including the purchase of the pig. It's a little more now, I have yet to see how much more. I know the cost of the pig had doubled since the last time we bought pigs. We couldn't raise any pigs for a few years and this year we have four to make up for lost time I suppose. I'll refigure all the costs again at the end of this season and see what difference is.

Our plan was to raise hogs every other year when we started. Now we are leaning more toward having at least two every year now. I have been out of bacon for quite some time now, if I am complaining about that it's because I so love bacon! I would rather raise only one hog every year and maybe two every other year. I have a feeling that the one hog would be too lonely by itself. So we'll probably stay with having at least two hogs at a time. They are very intelligent and social creatures. We think it would be an unhappy hog if it were raised all by its lonesome.

Hogs are so very smart. I swear they are little genius's. As they get bigger and taller, they find ways to open gate latches and all kinds of other silly things. After our first few hogs we began to realize that you have to treat them like small mischievous little children. Genius small children even. Everything in and around the hogs must be childproofed. Much the same way as you would child proof a kitchen to keep small children from getting into things they aren't supposed to be into. Just the same as keeping them in certain rooms so you can keep an eye on them. Hogs are no different in my opinion. If you have a gate that you don't want them to figure out, then you may not want to operate the latch in front of them more than once or twice, if you do, they'll learn how to open it. You'll learn quickly a better way to lock it or to use a keyed lock.

Anytime we bring new hogs home we always introduce them to our dogs. That way the dogs realize that the hogs are now a part of our little farm family and they will protect them as well. The dogs will bark if something comes in toward the hog pen just as they will when something is headed for the chicken coop. Also, it seems to be the polite thing to do. The dogs will usually run around the pen with them and play with them and bark at them at first. It is so hilarious when the pigs bark back and wag tails as the dogs do. It only took a couple minutes and one of the hogs was imitating our little beagle. Running and playing around as she does. Hogs are a lot of fun to have around. You never know what to expect next.

The very first time we went to pick up our first pigs was so much fun. The farmer we bought them from was pretty cool. He answered a bunch of questions for all of us. We were letting a friend raise a couple hogs at our place so we all met at the farmers place to get the pigs. Even funnier to me was that fact that our friends girlfriend can't stand the smell of a farm, add to that a pig farm and I couldn't quit laughing. The farmer showed us around a bit and asked if we wanted to hold a baby pig. Of course I did, baby animals are so adorable. Baby pigs are so darn cute! I will tell you this, that farmer did that on purpose so he could get a laugh because he already knew. You can't hold the little buggers! If they squirm, good luck because they are nothing but muscle. I could not believe how strong a three week old pig is! Hell, I still can't believe it. I was all worried about hurting the little pig, I didn't want to drop it, so I was trying to hurry up and hand it back before it got loose. They were all laughing at me. That is what I call good clean fun!

When we all got our hogs we ended up with four for ourselves and two for our friends. That was my first year ever having hogs, so I learned a lot that year. First and foremost I learned not to operate gate latches around smart little piggy's.

On another occasion I had to call the farmer back to ask him a question about one of the hogs. I guess he wasn't technically a hog, he was a neutered male. He had been acting funny and walking a little sideways. At any rate, when I talked to the farmer I wasn't paying any attention to the fact that I was in a dollar store at the time and referring to our pig as the name we had given him; Pork Chop. I was more concerned with making sure Pork Chop was ok and I didn't care where I was or who was listening. It took a minute or two for the farmer to quit laughing and I was laughing too because he was and saying "what"? No one could believe I was serious and had named him Pork Chop. All the pigs got names, but everybody loved Pork Chop. He had told me that Pork Chop probably had water in his ear and as long as nothing looked bad that he would probably be fine and we would most likely not have to call a vet. He was right, no vet was needed and Pork Chop ended up getting the water out of his ear a few days later and was fine.

Back to lesson number one. Our first gate was a chain link gate like you would normally see around a house with a chain link fence I guess. The kind where the latch gets lifted up to open the gate. One that you could use a padlock on if you needed to lock the gate. Using a padlock didn't make sense then, I didn't want to hunt for keys every time I needed to get into the hog pen. I used a piece of aluminum that was left over from putting up the fence. Those aluminum fence ties I think they are, whatever it is I thought it would work and be easy enough to get in and out of the pen. I put it through the padlock hole on the gate and had it in almost a circle. It just barely needed to be bent to be able to undo it. A hogs snout didn't look to me like it would be able to squeeze into the small gap between the fence post and the gate to unravel the aluminum piece I had put there to keep them from lifting the gate handle. Apparently that snout was not only able to go there, but was also able to remove the piece of aluminum as well.

We were outside and Joseph had spotted some tracks behind the house. We have a lot of deer around here so at first glance that's what he thought it was. I remember him saying these are funny looking deer tracks back here honey. I had started to walk over to where he was and it hit him, these are not deer tracks, they are hog tracks! Uh oh!

Sure enough when I ran back around to the other side of the house and to the hog pen the door was wide open and there were no hogs. At this particular point in time the hogs were already scheduled for slaughter at the end of that week. We only had two left and they were gone for the season. We followed the tracks through the woods and next door to the neighbors horse pasture. There they were. The neighbor wasn't home, and I was in a panic. Not only to try to keep the pigs from hurting anything, but to not lose our hogs either. We had a lot of time and money invested in these guys. If we were going to have to lose any hogs, now was not the best time to lose them. Joseph tried to steer them out of the neighbors horse pasture area and away from the yard toward the road, and so did I. The two pigs kept running around and playing, but were not having any part of letting us get close enough to try to catch them. I don't know what we were thinking, because we were running around trying to catch them and we had nothing to catch them with. No rope, no food, no nothing. Joseph left to get a rope and some food, which I hadn't noticed at the time because I was too busy hoping for damage control and chasing the pigs around. Not only that but he hadn't said anything to me before he took off.

As if things weren't already funny enough, the pigs ran up to the neighbor's garage door and that is where they wanted to stay. I would chase them back toward the road, which I guess I should clarify that we live on a dead end dirt road with little traffic. So no I wasn't running them toward a busy black-topped road or anything. Each time I would run them away from the garage they would do a circle and go right back. During all of these circles we were doing I was able to get a little closer to the hogs each time. Finally I managed to step in between them and they began to walk with me. I had one hand on the back of each hogs ear, scratching the back of their ears as you would a dog. We started walking together, and they were getting distracted by everything they seen. When they would start to wander away from my side towards the woods I would just scratch a little harder and talk to them. I was telling them what sweet little cute piggy's they were. I had one hog on each side of me, and we had made it to the road. It's kind of a long way from where I managed to catch up with the pigs to our house and the hog pen.

Once the hogs and I made it to the road they tried to veer off into the woods. I just kept saying good sweet little piggy's and scratching their ears, and trying my hardest to be the lead hog and hoping they would follow. As I was walking down the middle of the road with the hogs in tow, Joseph came around the side of the house with a rope in his hand and spotted me first.

He yelled to me that he had a rope, but I wasn't going to say a word. I did not want anything to screw up leading the hogs as far as I had managed to get them at that point. I just kept scratching and say they were good little piggy's and shaking my head no at the same time at Joseph. At first he looked confused. Then as he got a little closer he seen the hogs and immediately shut up and stepped back. I was keeping my steps at a steady pace and I was not about to stop scratching or saying good little piggy's because it was working and they were still following along with me.

At this point I was thinking that with my luck a car will be coming down the road at any moment and that we are going to lose our hogs. Joseph isn't sure what to do, or if he should try to do anything at all. As I turned the hogs into the driveway and began to head to the hog pen it was everything I could do not to laugh. The hogs stayed right with me all the way up until I got within about twenty feet of their pen. From there they ran ahead of me and went back into the pen on their own. The first thing that came out of Josephs mouth after the gate was closed was "how the hell did you do that"? Like I knew. I had no idea why they had followed me home. I told him that would likely never happen again and I was just glad the hogs were home and back in the pen.

The adrenaline had subsided and we were both saying I can't believe we got them back. We were laughing so hard at all the possibilities that could have taken place and the fact that for once things had gone our way. Could you just imagine the look on someone's face if they had driven down our road that day? How hilarious would I, and our hogs, have looked walking right down the middle of the road together? I wish we could have videotaped that, it was such an unbelievable set of events. All I can say about that is if our hogs weren't very happy with their home and us, things most likely would have turned out quite differently that day.

Joseph and I learned at a young age that many farm animals are around for a single purpose and that you should never get attached to them. That is all fine and well, but why can't their short lived existence be enjoyable? Why can't I enjoy them while they are around? Well, that is how I see it anyway, and so does Joseph. This year we haven't named any of the hogs, I think we ran out of cute names. When they hear; "where's my piggy's?", they come running. I used to think they just enjoyed someone scratching their noses, now I think they are frisking you for a hand out. Much like the dogs do sniffing for where the treat went or whose pocket it is in. We usually take lots of pictures of them as they are growing and we will spend what time we can in the pen with them and play with them sometimes. They seemed to enjoy the old basketball we threw in there, they would bat it around sometimes. They used to anyway, until one chomped on it and deflated it. My answer to that was to get a bigger ball, one they can't get their teeth into. I bought one of those giant kick balls. It was like two feet tall from the ground up. My answer was wrong, that ball didn't last long either before they popped it too. They seem to be quite content playing with the branches that fall into the pen as well as the deflated basketball. It is so funny to see a pig run by with a big stick in its mouth. Makes me want to yell fetch! Like I said, they always end up acting just like the dogs. My only complaint about raising hogs is the extra flies that begin to hang around the house in the summer. Other than that I rather enjoy having them around.

Yesterday when I went in the hog pen to feed the four hogs we have now, they are getting ornery. We had to up the amount of food because they were starting to stay hungrier. The biggest hog started jumping around and barking at me. I was kind of in a hurry and was wearing sandals so I didn't hang around long. I had asked Joseph if he had heard the one hog barking at me and he said he did. He reminded me that the hogs like it when you run with them and play with them like you'd play with your dog. Next time I go in to feed them I'll have to be prepared to play a little. I'd try a Frisbee if I knew they wouldn't try to eat it.

When the hogs get closer to butcher weight we set up an appointment with someone who will haul them to the butcher for us. There are a couple of different guys that have cattle trailers that will come and pick up your hogs, and take them to the butcher for a fee. That works out great because we don't have a cattle trailer, and they are inexpensive enough that it is easier for us to use their services as opposed to buying a trailer just for that purpose.

You ain't had bacon or sausage until you have raised it from a youngin' and had it butchered with a company that will give you back your meat. It doesn't even cook the same as that crap you buy from the store. It took me a month to learn how to cook *real* meat after we got our first hogs back from the butcher. You can eat whatever you want, but I have no intentions of ever eating bacon or sausage from the store ever again. I would sooner starve or live off of road kill first. Yes, I mean that! If you think the meat you're getting from the store is good, try some real down home farm raised meat and then tell me what it is you think you're eating from the stores. If you want to argue with me then, I'll have no choice but to tell you that you have removed your taste buds and that I am sorry for your shitty luck.

If you doubt me, then test me and my theory by finding a farmer that will allow you to purchase a portion of a steer or a hog that has been raised the right way and not for sale to a store. I wish you luck in finding one at the rate that we are allowing our farmers to be pushed out of the mainstream. If you are lucky you'll be in an area where all of the farmers haven't been shoved out the main stream door just yet. Maybe a place where all the new city people moving into the country haven't started complaining about the smell yet. Take my opinion for what it is, my opinion. I'm just sick and tired of watching the farms disappear and no-one seems to be doing jack about it. We need our farms and our farmers. I hope you realize that and work to support the farmers any way you possibly can. By from local farmers and farmers markets when you can. I know we are all in a bind, but what will we do without our back bone in our food industry? Think. Do you want to eat liquid smoke covered bacon from the store or real food from real farmers in your community?

In all seriousness though, raising your own food is the best for you in every respect. To not waste anything we get back from our hogs is a good feeling. If we were able to butcher our own hogs, we would use even more. That is a job we have not yet tried to do ourselves. There are only so many hours in a day, I think we are pushing the limits as it is. Choosing to do a little farming if you have the area promotes a healthier life style. You'll no longer have to worry about recalls when food has been improperly handled because you'll know exactly where it came from. You might end up learning a few new things and you might have a little fun in the process.

Chapter 14
Hog Stories

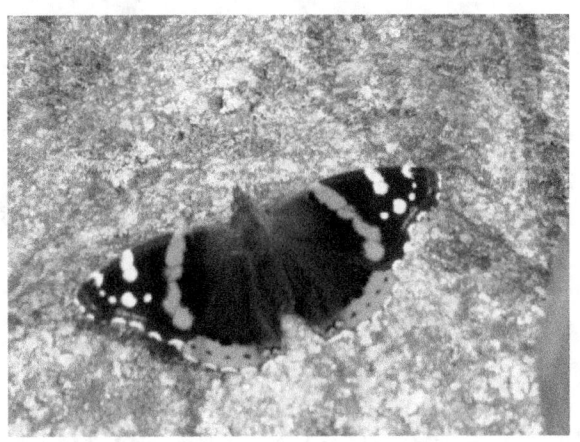

{This is a picture of a butterfly taking a break on one of the boulders next to the flowers.}

I was always under the impression that hogs would eat greens, roots, and grubs. Things they would graze and root around to eat. I hadn't really put much thought into hogs eating much else.

In the summer months we tend to feed our chickens less than we do in the winter time for obvious reasons. The chickens can get out and hunt for bugs, which is much better for them anyway. Chickens are also smart when they want to be. They know how to find easy food. Easy food would be in the hog pen. Hog food is really powdery which I can't stand because so much gets wasted, but it is what it is I guess. When the hogs start getting bigger we start feeding them twice a day to make sure they are getting enough food to get them up to weight in time for when we like to ship them to the butcher.

We won't use supplements or anything to promote growth, just the feed mix we buy from the store that we're told has no steroids or anything in it. Back to my point here. When the hogs get fed twice a day, it is not uncommon for quite a bit of food to be left over and sit around all afternoon. Once the chickens realize that extra food is just laying around in there, they look for ways to get into it and eat it. Some of our chickens are miniatures and they fly really well. The other chickens are regular size and aren't very good fliers. Keeping the mini chickens out of anywhere is pretty much impossible if they want in where ever that might be. I was sitting on the porch watching the garden for ground hogs when I heard a huge ruckus going on by the hog pen. It sounded like something had gotten hold of a chicken and was killing it or dragging it off into the woods. Around here we have many elements to watch out for when the chickens are out. It is not uncommon to see a coyote, cat, dog, or opossum running off into the woods with a chicken. We try to be at the ready for anything at virtually any time of day. You can't be everywhere all the time though.

When I rounded the corner at the chicken coop to investigate I couldn't see anything in the woods but I could hear that chicken squawking. I ran further to see around the pig hut to the back of the hogs pen and watched the final gulp of a chicken going down the hogs throat. I had heard similar to what I had just heard over the past weeks, but each and every time I investigated I would find nothing. No evidence and no feathers, just nothing. The hog ate the chicken! What amazed me as much as that was the fact there was not a single feather left to be a clue as to where that chicken had gone. If I had not seen that hog eating that chicken I wouldn't have known what had just happened. The chickens are always carrying on a clucking when they lay an egg or when they see a bird fly over head, so I'm used to those types of squawks.

The next day the very same thing happened again. Only this time I knew where to go to and thought I would be able to save this chicken from being eaten. The hogs were chasing the chicken around the pen, and apparently the chicken panicked and forgot it could fly out, it was a mini. I tried to get between them but the hogs ran right on over me, literally, and snatched that chicken up and ate it before I could do anything about getting back on my feet or getting my balance back. I am not sure just how many chickens we lost to that group of hogs, but I know it was at least a few. The fence around our hog pen is about ten foot high chain link fencing. When we we're finished putting it up I never dreamed anything would be able to get out of it, let alone get into it.

Here not too long ago we we're outside and heard the chickens making a fuss and when Joseph rounded the corner to the hog pen to check it out he got a big surprise. There was a coyote trying to dig its' way into the hog pen to get at the hogs. When I said that we have to be ready for anything at virtually any time of the day or night, I wasn't kidding. When Joseph started toward the coyote to scare it off, it left, but it wasn't in a particularly big hurry to leave. I have seen many things around here, but definitely did not expect to see a coyote digging into the hog pen while pretty much doing so right in front of us. While we were walking around and talking within forty feet of that enclosure. That seems a little to brave for my liking.

When I was growing up I was taught that if you see a coyote or a raccoon out before dusk or in the middle of the day that it was most likely sick. Sick apparently meant it had rabies. Anytime I have ever seen a critter like that out in the middle of the day, it has truly looked sick. We always have a gun handy in case it's needed, you never know. I'm pretty sure I can't out run a coyote, nah…I'm really sure! I know it can't outrun a bullet. So far we have had no real incident with the hogs and the coyotes, and I hope it stays that way. I'm not keen on the idea of shooting a coyote simply because it is trying to get at the pigs. I would much prefer that everyone survives and that we can manage to co-habitate together if at all possible. Even though I have a gun ready to use, I will always try to run it off first. As long as it isn't sick, it will go and we all win.

One year we were shipping a couple hogs in to the butcher first, because they were they only two out of the six or seven we had that were the right weight to go. Feeding hogs when they get close to slaughter weight can get fairly expensive, and not fun for me because I'm small. It would be like a Yeti thinking it can play with an ant and not hurt it; highly unlikely. That's how the pigs get with me as they get bigger. They mean well, but they are just too big for playing like they want to. So as soon as they are ready to go, it's off to the butcher with them. When we built the hog pen we weren't exactly thinking about having to separate hogs to wrestle them into a cattle trailer. A couple of pieces of thick fencing and a piece of plywood and some screws were all we could come up with to try to help this fiasco along. This goes back to what I said in the beginning of this book about always plan for anything, you need to be creative about what the possibilities could end up being with anything you venture into.

I'm going to guess that our hog pen is about fifteen yards long by about maybe ten yards wide. Give or take a little, but I'm not that far off I don't think. What truly makes this funny is the time of year it was and the weather that year. It was fall and we had a monsoon season that year. I think it rained all summer and all winter that year. The hog pen was so soupy you could barely walk in to feed them twice a day. Picture six hogs, Joseph, and myself in a pen with muck that in some areas you could sink almost to your knees in. When I say muck, I really mean wet and sticky pig shit in a muck pit. Now try to imagine how we are going to cut two hogs out of that herd, keep the other four in check, and get the two that need to go into the cattle trailer. Word of advice, when planning any adventure, think about *all* of the possibilities that will arise later.

Somehow we managed to get several hogs to into their pig hut. A little ten foot by ten foot enclosure we built for their shelter. I hurried and drove some screws through the plywood to block the door and to hopefully contain the hogs long enough to load the two that needed to go. These hogs were very happy to be together and did not want to be separated. The "lead" hog was one of the hogs I had locked in the pig hut. Need I say the "lead" hog was the biggest? The piece of plywood I had available only covered three quarters of the door. There was still about a foot or two at the top that was open. The one lead hog kept trying to jump up to see what was going on and I knew it was only a matter of time before that hog ripped down the plywood.

In the meantime, Joseph and I are trying to run around and corral the hogs out the gate. They wanted no part of leaving, the gate, or any part of the trailer. I chained a sturdy piece of fencing to the chain link fence where the gate was, and this extra piece of fencing was just long enough to make it to the corner of the pig hut. We thought we had made a chute for the hogs and that we could run them into the trailer with it. Wrong. There was no way I could hold that fencing up when that hog decided it was going through it and not into that trailer. As if it wouldn't be bad enough to attempt this circus when it was dry in the hog pen, this was hilarious! After the first time that hog ran through my fabricated pig chute, I was completely covered in shit. Literally. Not only did I fall down in it, when the pig ran past me it sprayed me with liquid shit again. We went at this approach for every bit of an hour and a half if not two hours.

During this time, the older gentleman who had the cattle trailer and the appointment with us to pick our hogs was being a very good sport through all of this. He must have had plenty of time, or just knew from talking to us that this was our first time doing this. He was standing at the fence and laughing as much as he was trying to give us advice on how to get those hogs in the trailer. He said he would help us any way he could, but he had no intentions of stepping into the super sized muck/shit mess that was in that pen. We completely understood his point on that one! If I was him, I wouldn't have gotten in there either. He was such a kind and very patient man who must have had some funny stories for his grandkids after leaving our house!

We eventually got the hogs in the trailer with one extra that wasn't supposed to go. I had never seen the inside of a cattle trailer before and didn't know all the doors moved here and there to make separating the animals quite a lot easier. He moved a few gates around and out ran the one that wasn't supposed to go. We apologized I don't know how many times to that man for all of the chaos. He was such a good sport through it all. After that Joseph and I went back to our drawing boards to devise a better plan to run the hogs into a trailer in the future. We took the advice of the ever so patient man that hauled our hogs for us that day as well.

When he once again returned to haul another several hogs for us, I think he was pleased to see the new chute that we had made to make things easier and quicker for all of us. He still laughed at me though, and quite honestly I can't blame him. I can be easily frustrated and I'm quite small framed, so it must be pretty funny to watch hogs run me over and me get back up madder than a hornet and go after them again. Hell I'd laugh too!

He really got a kick out of me trying to bribe the hogs into the trailer with peanut butter cookies. I was dead serious about it. They would follow me anywhere if had cookies, so why would this day be any different? Joseph was irritated by my silliness and told me I sounded like a moron and not to embarrass him. The very patient man thought it was funny though. My argument was a simple "what will it hurt to try"? Stranger things happen around our house on a daily basis, you never know until you try right? I am silly enough to try just about anything once, twice if it works. It didn't work, and the hogs could've cared less what kind of a treat I had in my hand that day. At least I eliminated another possibility from my crazy list of things I think are possible that I have in my head. Besides, people who are too worried about how silly they will look if they try something new, will never discover anything new. At least we all got to laugh. Laughing is very good for your soul, do it often.

Chapter 15
Nothing Wasted

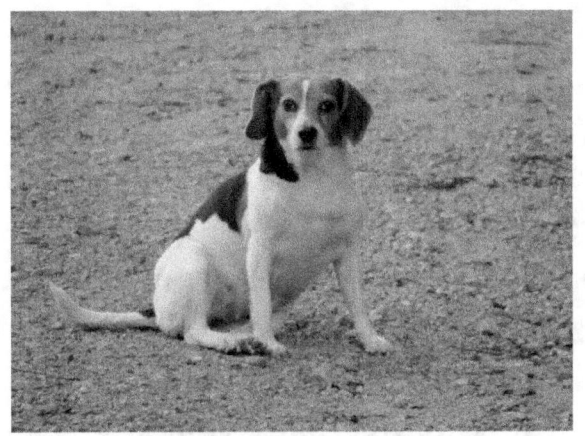

{This is my fussy little supervisor again, she is such a character!}

Whether you have a big farm or a small farm you will not have to waste anything. When the hogs are in season, they get all of the table and garden scraps. When the hogs are gone the garden and table scraps are split between the dogs and the chickens.

I was told by a farmer in my travels that if you raise hogs to sell for human consumption that feeding them table scraps is strictly prohibited. Apparently due to a disease that broke out in Europe I think many, many years ago. I guess they had attributed this outbreak to table scraps somehow. At any rate that was news to me. We don't sell our hogs so we don't care. We know where everything comes from around here and it has never been a problem for us. Like I said, we do things how they work for us and very rarely do we listen to what anyone other than a farmer tells us is good or bad.

For a while it was said that people shouldn't eat eggs, then all of the sudden they are good for you again. I have always known eggs are good for you because they are natural. If we can grow it or raise it, then we know it is good. One of the joys of living like we do is that we can eat anything we want because we work hard. By anything we want I don't mean fast food or junk food, I mean the food we grow or harvest when hunting seasons are in or the garden is coming in.

No matter what somewhere, somehow, some body around here can and will benefit from each and everything that is grown and harvested on our land. It just depends on what part of the season we are in for who gets the most from what.

Right now the pigs are getting everything, and in another three months the dogs and the chickens will get everything. No matter how you view it, someone is always getting treats and we are never having to waste anything. How can things get any better than that?

Hunting is a natural part of life's cycle. We hunt ethically, only for what we need and not status or bullshit bragging rights. Two simple rules to live by for us are to hunt justly and in tune with the natural order of things. This means that selfishness does not become part of the equation.

When the garden is finished the hogs get all of the plants we pull up. If they are plants they like that is. What the hogs don't eat, the chickens will pick at. If we aren't raising hogs that year then the chickens and the deer get all of the gardens left over's. When I am picking vegetables in the garden I always find at least a few tomatoes or peppers or whatever else that a bug has been eating on. I always carry an extra basket for anything that the pigs or chickens should get. On my way back to the house to unload the baskets I stop off and dump a basket to either the hogs or chickens, or sometimes both.

I don't believe in city ordinances, if you have enough room to raise anything it is you want to eat, you should be allowed by law to do so. Screw your city neighbors that should have stayed in the city if they didn't like the country. Screw them any ways if you live in the city. Why should you suffer because your neighbors are grocery store loving idiots who are too prissy to handle smelling an animal that reeks of purity and goodness for your body. As long as you can provide a reasonable environment for the livestock you want to raise, you should be able to.

I know I mentioned it before but I was growing tomatoes on my balcony when I was living in an apartment. I can only be without real produce for so long before I start looking for ways to make it happen. I am just thankful that Joseph and I are so much alike. Our deck and flower beds have vegetable plants and herbs growing them each year. We have pumpkins that have almost spanned the entire one side of our house and will soon be into the flower beds. Does that make us look like hicks? I'm not sure, but I know I don't care if it does. We utilize every inch of available space in the best way possible.

It should be a God given right to eat off the land as nature had originally intended and as my ancestors did before me no matter where I may live. I wish more people would think ahead and stop clearing land for over development and leave some of nature in the process of their need to build and squeeze every last penny out of our natural world at the cost of our environment and its inhabitants. I also wish leaving enough habitat for wildlife would always be a consideration when planning new developments, along with leaving wetlands intact.

I miss our country, when things were real and when the farmers got the respect they deserve, not the shaft every time they turn around. When ignorant people weren't crying about the smell or the view. If you don't like farm country, then don't move there. No matter who you are remember that without our farmers we'll be dependent on other countries or other sources for food. The thought of not being able to be self sufficient should bother more people than it seems to in my opinion. Nothing compares to the taste and the nutritional value of *real* food.

I know I have mentioned this before, but Joseph and I both have strong Native American Indian roots. For us it is very important to not waste things. Anything from electricity and water to food, we conserve what we can and use no more than we need. On the average we put out no more than one smaller sized bag of trash per week with four people living in our home. Now that we have found a recycle program through or trash collector, many times isn't even that one small bag anymore. I have called our trash company on more than one occasion and told them not to send the garbage truck down our road because we have no trash to set out this week, and that I see no need in them wasting the fuel and the time to drive all the way down our road for nothing.

When you can your food and reuse the jars it produces no waste. Even though canning jar lids cannot be used twice I save them all anyway. I have used them for a number of different things. One of those uses was to attach them to strings and hang them around the garden. They make noise when they bang together and they have worked similar to a scarecrow, only better. There are many things that get thrown away everyday that could be used for something other than just filling a landfill. The lids are made of metal and could even be taken to a scrap yard. We try to think of everything, and hold off on throwing many things away until we either figure out a second use for them or figure out a way they can be recycled. Caring for Mother Earth is our first thought in any decision we make or anything we do.

When we bought a slew of tomato cages for the garden and realized that the tomatoes grew too tall and broke off, we didn't throw them away. They sat in a pile for a year or two, then I started using them for green beans and peas. They work well for that, I was very happy we didn't waste them and that we had found a good use for them. We may have several piles of different things around the house, and even though I don't like having piles of things around, it eventually gets reused or hauled out for scrap. I can handle the piles if that means less is going to landfills, and less waste is being created.

Joseph recently got creative and made one of the most beautiful trellis' for our flowering vines that I have ever seen. He made the entire trellis from scrap out of one of the piles. The pile got smaller and he added beauty to the yard and flowers with a one of a kind trellis. Each time one of us is able to accomplish something like that it makes us both feel really good about all of the things we do. It reminds us all the time how lucky we are to live where we do and be able to do the things we do every day. We are blessed in every way to be able to enjoy the natural world around us and we never allow ourselves to take that for granted or to abuse it. It is a passion of ours to respect that blessing and make the best use of everything without damaging it and without taking from it anything more than we need.

Chapter 16
Farm Life

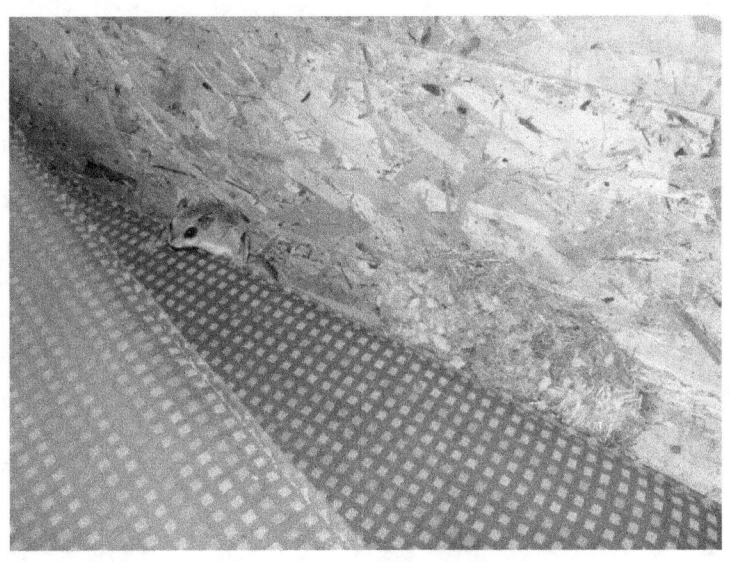

{This is a picture of a flying squirrel who had babies in our deer blind. If you look close you can see the nest that contains her babies to the right of her.}

Living in the woods is completely different than living in a city. Though we are surrounded by the city, our property is mostly wooded. Anytime we leave to run to the store or go to work there is a huge difference once we reach the edge of our property.

It's always hotter down the road. Being surrounded by cement and usually lacking too many trees, the city is always warmer than the wooded areas. Trees are like natural air conditioners and emit cooler air. I don't believe this is simply because they provide shade. Being under an umbrella doesn't provide a cooler atmosphere around it, but trees do. When we take walks through the woods on hot summer evenings, I usually make sure to grab a flannel shirt to take with me, because on many occasions I come back with goose bumps. It gets chilly out in the woods, even when it is eighty degrees and humid. The woods have a tendency to be damp as well. Everything else can be dry, but out in the woods it's usually cool and somewhat damp. Yes, this can and usually does mean more mosquitoes as well as mold. I'll fight with the mosquitoes in the country any day as compared to living where there is little left of the natural world.

This will probably sound funny to some, but makes a lot of sense to others like us. Joseph and I haven't frequented the bars to play pool much since about the first or second year we were together. We both very much enjoy playing pool, and we used to do so all the time. As a matter of fact that is how we met, I had been playing pool on a local pool league. Joseph and I ended up in a conversation one evening and from there we became friends for quite a while before we started dating. Once we began gardening, canning, and raising livestock we got really busy.

Between working fifty or more hours a week, we were also putting in hours around our small farm that felt like a second full time job. We began running out of time to play pool, or socialize with our friends. We couldn't really afford to be going out anyway, buying feed for the animals gets expensive. Though we were working a lot and probably could have used more nights out, it just wasn't feasible. I would venture to say that in the last four or five years we have gone out maybe twice. We have gone out to dinner here or there for birthdays a few times, but for the most part that isn't very enjoyable anymore. Not after eating as healthy as we usually do on a daily basis. It has become more pleasurable for us to stay home and enjoy watching our garden grow and spending time together making a real home grown meal. Animals of all kinds are many hours of free entertainment, especially when you live in the woods.

A few months ago Joseph and I had about fifty dollars and I was itching for the first time in probably four or five years to go shoot a game or two of pool. We headed out and went to one of the only bars close to us to shoot pool. We don't like to venture far on Friday or Saturday nights or any other night for that fact. I can't stand being in a car for any length of time. I hate sitting still that long I guess, all I know is I don't like driving anywhere I don't have to. Once we got there and rented our pool table we were laughing about how much we used to enjoy these nights out. Now that we were there and were actually playing pool, it just wasn't as much fun as we had remembered it being to hang out in a bar. We didn't really want to have more than a beer or two, because we wanted to make sure we had enough time before we left to drive home and to be completely sober. There wasn't a whole lot of people in the bar, which I was quite happy about. I'm not much for crowds, never really have been actually. I like my personal space un-invaded. It's funny because Joseph is the way I am when it comes to that issue. We had been there a about an hour I guess and we ordered a second beer. The plan was that we would stay long enough after that beer to be sure we were good to drive home. We were going to play one more game of pool and then turn the pool balls in and sit and talk before we left. We were playing our last game of pool when Joseph and I looked up and a second other pool table was being claimed by another group of people. It was about this time that we both spotted a mosquito buzzing around our table, and it would not leave us alone. I don't think we finished the last game of pool before we took the pool balls back to the counter. Neither one of us could even play because we kept watching where that flying dirty needle was going and swatting at it. By that time all we could do was watch for it, we barely talked with the exception of wondering who's blood was already on that damn thing and wondering if they had any diseases. If a mosquito can bite a certain kind of mouse and then bite a horse and give that horse a strain of a flu virus that can also be passed to humans. Not only be passed to humans, but responsible for several deaths as well. No-one can tell me that a mosquito won't pass other diseases too. In a target rich environment I was not going to participate in sharing that dirty little flying needle. We had to get out of there. We left the bar and went and stood around in the parking lot for a while before we left for home. I looked at Joseph and told him that I had remembered why we had more fun staying at home than we did going out anymore. Call me paranoid and I won't rightly care, I cannot handle facing a mosquito bite anywhere but in the woods.

I have been taking my chances sharing the dirty needles with the animals for years. The way I see it, my chances are far better at avoiding aids and who knows what else out here in the woods and I like it that way just fine.

It sort of bugs me when the people we know are always telling us that we need to go out more, get away from the house more often because we need a break now and then. I'll take my break when I'm ready, and I'll do it where I am happiest, in the woods. I don't understand why people just don't get it. Taking a break from work and wandering around the woods for a couple hours is exactly what I not only need, but greatly enjoy. Being out in the woods makes me feel better both emotionally and physically. Especially when I am blessed enough to have an encounter with any wild animal. Those moments are priceless to me. If we go anywhere else we are always miserable with it in the end anyway.

People are always selfish and in such a hurry that they are rude to everyone else around them. Whether it's in a car or in an establishment. Society has become so selfish and stuck to cell phones that most people only care about what they are doing and care nothing for what or who is around them. When we walk through the woods the air is so much cleaner and fresher. It is invigorating and a good work out as well. We always feel better after we've been home for a few minutes after we have gone to the city. There is nothing like the smell of the fresh country air filling your lungs with air that is way cleaner than you'll find in any city, whether the city is big or small. The trees filter the air and the difference is very noticeable, even to friends of ours when they come over most times. Many people comment on how much cooler and cleaner it feels around our house. How calming the quiet and the flower beds are. How cool it is to hear the birds chirping and going to and from the feeders. I fail to see the logic of trading that for the city and calling it fun.

I guess maybe people who have been raised in a city might not understand how we could find farm life better than city life. It is kind of the same thing as vegetarians and people with or without tattoos. I seen a little poster once that said the only difference between tattooed people and non-tattooed people is the fact that tattooed people don't care if you have a tattoo. The same concept seems to follow hand in hand with a great many other kinds of people as well.

Of all the people we come into contact with, be it friends or strangers when we are out somewhere. We seem to be the only ones not telling other to people to move to a farm, start eating meat, start hunting, and the like. Everyone always thinks they should tell us what will make our lives happier or more politically correct in one way or another. It would be an ideal world if people would mind their own business more. If they would put all of the energy they use telling other people how to live into fixing their own families and lives at home. I know we do.

Yesterday was Saturday and we spent our afternoon gathering firewood for this coming winter. When we were finished we had a garden fresh salad and we were stuffed. After working outside Joseph enjoys relaxing to a good movie. I don't mind watching movies, but I do have a hard time sitting still that long most of the time. He is always telling me to learn to relax. I just love to go and I have trouble slowing or stopping. Maybe that is why farm life fits with me so well, maybe I am geared for it. I have two speeds; high or off. Who knows, maybe working is my form of relaxation, or maybe sleep is. I have heard lots of people comment that weeding a flower bed is how they relax. Weeding a flower bed is work though, maybe I am not alone on that one.

Another thing that Joseph and I started doing recently is making home-made wine. That has been so much fun! As it turns out there are several people we know that also make wine, we would have never guessed, because they are men. I don't mean that in a bad way by any means. In my mind I do not associate the words "men" and "wine" with any connection at all. Every man I have ever known either hated or at least didn't like wine and usually referred to it as a girl thing. Before we started to make wine ourselves, one of our friends had given us a bottle of his own wine to try. I opened it right away, because I have always liked wine. A good glass of wine with a salad or a steak is impossible for me to pass up. The bottle was almost gone and I kept pestering Joseph to try it. Finally he took this hilariously microscopic little drop for a taste, then sat there for a second. He looked confuzzled. He tasted again, only the next sip was a big one and his eyes lit up. He was completely surprised at just how different this wine was from any other he had ever been forced to try in the past. He was lucky he tried it when he did, because he got the last little glass that was left in that bottle. We washed the bottle out and returned it to the guy who had given it to us. He is the one who helped us get started making wine. He offered much advice and let me borrow books and helped us a great deal with little secrets and tricks to make better wine. Joseph was all over it, now he was picking out wine flavors to make and was right there helping and directing the entire way. He went from wine hater to wine maker and wine lover.

This last batch of wine we made was where he became a little to directive and should have just listened to me. There was too much liquid in one of the huge glass containers because he thought it should be full, when in actuality it wasn't supposed to be. I tried to tell him, but he wasn't listening. Okay I said, and let him fill the jar prematurely. I kind of knew what was going to happen, but I had no idea just how bad it was really going to be. I am not going to try to explain how to make wine here, but I will tell you that during the fermentation process the wine gets a little volatile.

That is normal, but you have to leave enough room in fermenter for the churning and swelling of its contents. This is where Joseph jumped to far ahead of himself and filled the jar. I kept watching it every day and wondering what was going to happen. One day we heard a loud noise in the dining room and it sounded like something had fallen over, it was kind of loud. We were looking around for what may have fallen off the wall or fallen over when a volcanic eruption was spotted. Towels now! The top had popped, no not popped-it *BLEW* off the jar. Not only did it spray the ceiling and walls at the initial blast of the top, it was spewing out the top and rolling like waves down the sides of the jar and going everywhere. I didn't know where to throw the first towel, or how I should even approach trying to contain this mess. I threw a towel and grabbed a cork and plugged the top and was trying to hold it there. Nope, there was so much pressure I couldn't contain it. It was so unbelievably funny, yet not so funny because I wasn't looking forward to figuring out how to clean it all up. It had finally spewed long enough that it had stopped overflowing everywhere. The mop up began. This is the point and time when Joseph listened when I was explaining that the jars need to have room for the contents to expand so things like this don't happen. We mopped and wiped up as much of the mess as we could and I moved the huge jar into the kitchen. This was red wine, and we now had a red speckled ceiling in our dining room. Red wine-white ceiling-ugh!

We both figured all would be good now and that enough room had been left to prevent future explosions. Wrong. A few days later I heard another loud noise coming from the kitchen, and that sound was strikingly familiar. I took off running for the kitchen and sure enough, it had exploded again and was once again spewing all over the place. In the kitchen is where we have a pellet stove. My stupid ass had put that jar right on top of the pellet stove. I threw a towel over the gap in the pellet stove where the electrical components are to stop the flow into that area, and once again tried to cork the darn thing. In the mean time I had been yelling for Joseph to come help because I was not letting loose of that cork until we moved the jar away from the pellet stove. With his help we move the jar and were able to prepare to slowly release the rest of the fluid and pressure that were coming out no matter what we tried to do to contain it. It finished spewing and we were once again back to mopping and wiping up. Now we had two white ceilings that were now covered in red wine polka dots. The walls came clean surprising easy just by wiping them down. Ceiling paint on the other hand is more like flat paint. Flat paint seems to soak things into it, and is virtually impossible to wipe or wash clean. You guessed it, our ceilings are still covered in red wine polka dots. I don't know how or why, because I am no wine expert, but that jar did that same thing two more times before we were done with it. At any rate, by then I was really rubbing in the fact that Joseph should have just listened to me in the first place. I can't say that it what started it for sure, but I knew I was going to use that for as many "I told ya so's" as I could! Sometimes a good I told you so or two can be a lot of fun. Well, when you aren't on the receiving end of it anyway.

We always have hilarious stories for our friends. There truly is never a dull moment around here. The joy of our lives is that we never know what to expect next. Be that good or bad.

Chapter 17
Remember How We Impact Where We Live

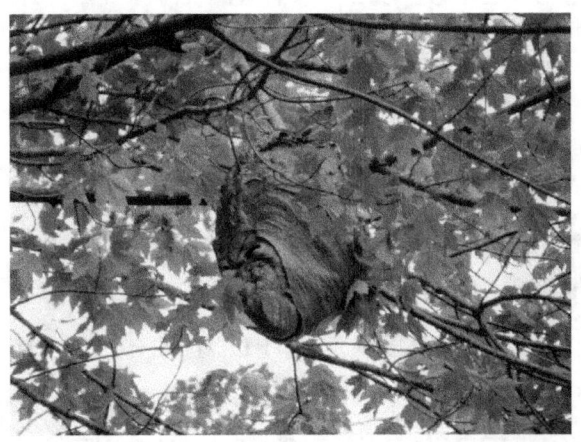

{This is a picture of a wasp nest that was in the front yard. Wow these ones are mean and aggressive.}

One chapter I really wanted to include in this book is this chapter. No matter who we are or where we live everything we do matters in one way or another. Doesn't matter if that impact at first is small or big, it will have residual effects that will follow in some way. All things are connected in some way shape or form.

All of the trash we put out must go somewhere in this world. An unfortunate truth is much of it gets sent to places who need the money and will accept your trash as long as you pay for them to take it. When these things go on in third world countries it can be devastating to their people and environments because their regulations aren't in place or enforced like those here in the U.S. because they usually have not found the need to contend with the types and amounts of waste the richer countries produce. That doesn't make what goes on behind closed doors right. It also doesn't mean that we as U.S. citizens should not care about the amount of trash we put out contributing to the problem. Everyone should at least make a small effort to recycle what they can and maybe even try to begin composting. Like I said, I am not going to stand on a soap box and tell people how they must live. I don't want anyone doing that to me, and I won't do that either. I do hope that making someone aware of the issues would at least make them think twice about even one thing that could be changed with little effort in their lives. We only have one planet. I just pray that it isn't too late to make positive enough impacts on our planet to keep it from puking us all out when it's had enough of our trash, contamination, and abuse. That or violent enough weather to wipe all of us out because the ecosystem has been knocked so far out of balance by so many not caring about taking care of our environment.

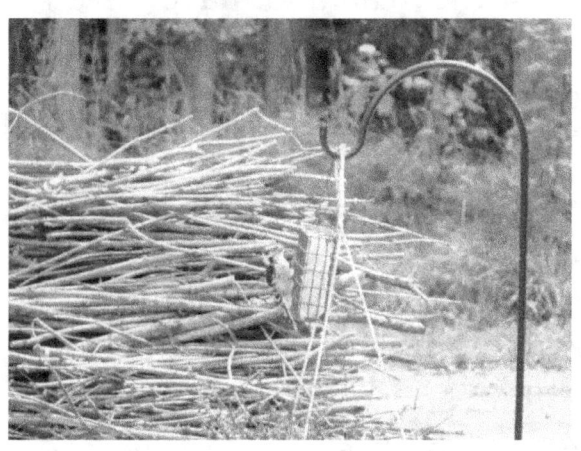

{This is a picture of a cute little woodpecker on one of our suet feeders.}

I'm no scientist but I do know that our planet will only continue with more and more violent weather the more our oceans and habitats are destroyed and polluted. The earths ecosystem and its beautifully fine tuned systems cannot take too much more before they all begin to deconstruct. If we as humans have negatively impacted enough of it and it can no longer support the next link of its intricate chain, then we're all screwed.

I wrote a poem about this when I was fifteen years old and it is now published in one of my poetry books called "A Collection of Poetic Expressions" and again in "Unspoken Truths: The Sad Reality". The poem is called "Greed" and I wrote it as I was watching the news about Prince Edward Sound and the Exxon Valdeez spill in my living room. That poem poured out of me in about as long as it took me to write it down. I was so upset to see the devastation man had inflicted on our environment. This year is 2010 while I am writing this book. I have been literally nauseous over feeling the hurt these oil spills and the habitat destruction have inflicted on nature. It hurts me when these things happen to our Earth. When the Exxon Valdeez spilled its oil I was also ill for a while during that as well. I still vividly see pictures of the ecosystem after the accident imbedded in my brain and etched in my heart. We only have one planet, and people can poke fun at green people all they want to, we need to consider the consequences of our actions ecologically, just as we have to on a societal level with legal matters, no matter what and no matter when. It is each individuals duty to do the right thing. I don't consider myself "green", I consider it my responsibility to care for the Earth I plan to live on for many more years. I don't want to use it all up for the generations to come to find nothing left but a big trash heap.

I don't care how much money anyone has. That does not give anyone the right to damage the planet or abuse its' resources. Or to take from me the wildlife habitat that supports the animals which allow me to support my way of life as my ancestors did.

This subject does not sit lightly with me and I take it very seriously being a hunter. I come from a very strong Native American back ground, and wish things could have been different many years ago. My ancestors spoke then of the damage to come by white men and the devastation that Mother Earth was yet to endure over all of the white man's endeavors. How did they know so much then? I believe they could feel it because they and the Earth and the nature around them were one and the same. If someone means you harm and they are near you, you should be able to sense and feel that. I have felt that pain for years and it weighs heavy in my heart and in my soul. We are all connected. I really hope more people learn how to fend for themselves and how to see the world around them. Not just as another place to find something to take from our Earth for money, but see the beautiful harmony around us for what it is. The delicate system which surrounds us that can only be turned upside down so many times before it implodes upon the human race. It is truly stupidity in destroying everything the Earth has to offer in the name of greed.

I know I have been one of the ones who aided in our Earth's destruction through foolish choices. We learn as we get older if we are not taught when we are young the impacts of our choices as we gain knowledge and begin to observe more of what is going on around us and in the world.

I have made a choice to pay closer attention to the smaller choices in life to make at least a small difference where I can. Choices as small as not buying a disposable water bottle or plastic cups all the time. Any little bit does matter and does make at least a small difference. If each person in our world makes a small difference it will add up very quickly to a very large impact in a positive way. I hope you will decide to make choices in your life through which you may be proud that you tried and have done what you can to take care of everything in and on our Earth within your means.

My only intention with adding this chapter is too make you aware of things that maybe you hadn't thought about before. Not to tell you how to live. Call if it food for thought. Call it anything you like, I just hope you realize the importance of preserving a world around us that will be able to sustain our population with food and livestock for protein. Without it we will not have much left with which to grow our own food and remain independent and healthier than those who chose big business to fill their freezers and cupboards.

From the Author

While I have been finishing this book it is fall. Our baby snapping turtles should have hatched by now. A couple days ago Joseph and I went to check on the eggs and Joseph pointed out that a mole had tunneled directly to the turtle eggs. I did not know that a mole would also eat eggs. I was so very sad when Joseph told me that we will not have baby snapping turtles again this year.

I have decided that if the turtle comes back this coming spring and lays her eggs again that I will dig them up. I am going to do what we did before that worked. I plan to put them in a cage in the yard and cover them with sand very close to where she lays the eggs. When we did that once before we had a one hundred percent success rate for the hatchlings, all fifty eggs hatched. We were able to carry fifty baby snapping turtles to the swamp that year. Hopefully we will be able to do that again next year.

Our hogs are scheduled to go in about four weeks and that timing couldn't be better because their appetites are eating our budget alive! We have once again been able to give thanks to those incredible animals for the blessings they provide us with. We have also been able to enjoy their company for yet another year. I'm sure the chickens will be glad when they go because they will once again get the scrap bucket for themselves.

Our garden is finished for the year with the exception of the pumpkins waiting to be carved. Though we didn't have as much success in the garden this year as I had hoped for. We still consider ourselves very blessed to able to have had the garden at all. Once again this year we learned many new things to try on next year's garden which will hopefully increase what we yield in the garden and what we are able to can and put away for the winter months. It's kind of funny to be outside with the squirrels preparing what we can for winter during the mid-summer and fall months. I guess we aren't all that much different from the squirrels after all. Especially when we are out gathering wood to keep ourselves warm through the winter months.

The deer have been finishing off the plants in the garden during the nights and mornings. I love being able to sit on the porch and watch them graze through the garden. Especially when the fawns are out there. They are such little spotted fire crackers. I love to watch them play and run around like they haven't a care in the world.

Not too long ago while Joseph and I were walking through the woods. We came across a very small dead fawn. Looking at the carcass that was left, it appeared that the coyotes had killed it.

Though I know that is how nature works, it is always a sad time for me when we lose one of the babies. I feel a special attachment to them. We have a few doe that stay close to our house. they will usually have their babies out back behind our house, and they tend to hang around back there while the fawns are young. Many times they have run in front of me while they are still wet after they were born. I feel greatly privileged that the doe trust us enough to keep their babies close to our home and us. At one point a doe allowed her twin babies to walk up to me. I'll save that story for another book, but that was an experience like nothing else I have ever known nor will I likely ever again experience.

I hope you have enjoyed the trip with me through our lives. I have enjoyed recapturing those moments in time and sharing them with you. I hope you have understood how we live our lives healthier than most and spend less money to do so. I hope you have realized that working for yourself in a garden or raising your own livestock can change your life in completely positive ways.

I hope you partake in the blessings of growing a garden if you are able and while you still can. Eat well and live well as nature and our ancestors before us intended.

More fiction and non-fiction books to look for by Shyanne Lee.

A Collection of Poetic Expressions

Twisted Love: The Evil Fed

Unspoken Truths

Fantosophy

Southern Flavor

Southern Grill & Game

Southern Garden Flavor

Books by Shyanne Lee can be found at www.amazon.com/books and type Shyanne Lee in the search box. Shyanne Lee can found at www.facebook.com by searching emailshyannelee@gmail.com.

www.ingramcontent.com/pod-product-compliance
Lightning Source LLC
Chambersburg PA
CBHW062124280526
45788CB00001B/40